# DOCTOR, WHY DOES MY FACE STILL ACHE?

# DOCTOR, WHY DOES MY FACE STILL ACHE?

## Getting Relief from Persistent Jaw, Ear, Tooth, and Headache Pain

by

Donald R. Tanenbaum, DDS, MPH

and

S. L. Roistacher, DDS

## *Gordian Knot Books*

An Imprint of Richard Altschuler & Associates, Inc.

New York

Distributed by University Press of New England
Hanover and London

3261668

Doctor, Why Does My Face Still Ache?: Getting Relief from Persistent Jaw, Ear, Tooth, and Headache Pain. Copyright © 2012 by Donald R. Tanenbaum and S. L. Roistacher. For information contact the publisher, Richard Altschuler & Associates, Inc., at 100 West 57th Street, New York, NY 10019, (212) 397-7233, or RAltschuler@rcn.com.

Library of Congress Control Number: 2011943449
CIP data for this book are available from the Library of Congress

ISBN-13: 978-1-884092-96-1

Gordian Knot Books is an imprint of
Richard Altschuler & Associates, Inc.

Cover Design: Josh Garfield

Printed in the United States of America

Distributed by University Press of New England
1 Court Street
Lebanon, New Hampshire 03766

# ACKNOWLEDGEMENTS

## Dr. Donald R. Tanenbaum:

As I embarked upon a career in dentistry in 1982, at what was then known as Columbia University School of Dental and Oral Surgery, little did I know that, almost 30 years later, I would be involved in one of the most exciting, stimulating and professionally rewarding areas of healthcare. The privilege of taking care of patients in pain is one that is not taken lightly, and not a day goes by that I don't in some way reflect on how fortunate I have been to have met so many giving professionals who either set me on or joined me on my ongoing journey.

A debt of gratitude must be extended to my friend and colleague Michael Gelb, DDS, who, with his simple question during my first year in dental school, "Do you want to hear my father lecture about TMJ?", gave me my first glimpse of what it would be like to dedicate a career to helping those in pain. With curiosity stimulated, Harold Gelb, DDS, opened my eyes and gave me the opportunity to see what life beyond dental school could be, if I was willing to be open minded, committed to excellence, and sensitive to the concerns and needs of patients, who would be putting their trust in my hands. His steadfast belief and insistence that I, as a dentist, could have a significant impact on the health and quality of life experienced by thousands of patients throughout my career, helped to shape the character and principles that pervade my practice today.

My relationship with my coauthor, S. L. Roistacher, DDS, began during a summer externship following my second year in dental school, and culminated in a dental residency that he directed at Queens Hospital Center in New York. This was the beginning of what is now a cherished friendship, built on shared interests and the love of learning. Dr. Roistacher's approach to teaching and patient care provided critical guidance, and his encouragement to pursue a career taking care of pain patients was instrumental in my career development. As the years passed, the idea of writing this book became a reality, and has allowed us to maintain a relationship built on mutual respect and the desire to care for those suffering with pain.

Special thanks must also be extended to Steven Graf-Radford, DDS, and Bernadette Jaeger, DDS, who were willing to share their knowledge and excitement as they were completing an orofacial training program at UCLA in 1983. Friendships along the way with Steve Syrop, DDS, Andy Kaplan, DDS, Steve Messing, DDS, and Matt Lark, DDS, continue to inspire excellence in all that I strive to achieve. My involvement and role as president of the American Academy of Orofacial Pain during 2009-2010 has also allowed me to associate with some of the finest clinicians, researchers and other people with whom I have shared the journey of my professional life. Thanks to all who have contributed to my professional development.

Not to be forgotten is unwavering enthusiasm from my family, who have shown remarkable support throughout my career and unlimited patience during the writing of this book. To my brother Robert L. Tanenbaum, PhD, who is a practicing clinical psychologist in Philadelphia, many thanks for your ideas, insights and countless re-reads and edits. The manuscript would never have been completed without your wisdom and advice. My three children, Natalie, Jenny and Betsy, continue to be a source of inspiration, as I make efforts to show them that through hard work and dedication anything is possible. To my wife, Cindy, thank you for keeping a smile on my face and reminding me that my greatest joy would be the journey of writing this book and not the end result. Lastly, I dedicate this book to the memory of my parents.

### Dr. S. L. Roistacher:

When I first announced to my wife that I had a book in me, her prompt response was, "Write it." However, neither of us knew that she would be at my side as I moved through the processing of many notes on paper and rough drafts to the finished product. Her support along the way was both encouraging and sustaining.

There are many people whom I would like to thank. Here are those who stand out. Each of them gave of their time and energy. Each had something different and special that I needed, if my efforts were to succeed. They are not listed in order of importance or intent. Without any one of them this book would never have been written.

1. Dr. Richard Schwimmer, MPH, DDS, a colleague and neighbor from time long past. He brought with him a broad range of experiences accumulated as associate director of the department of dental medicine in a large, local, voluntary hospital.

2. Geri Schwimmer, Coordinator for the Department of Dental Medicine at Queens Hospital Center, which I directed for over 20 years. In this role, she was the first contact potential patients had when they wished to see me. It was Geri who collected all of the data that I would have in advance of the first visit.

3. Toby Hobish, BS, PhD, a practicing psychologist who provided the understanding and insights I would need to take care of patients suffering with facial pain. Without her wisdom, the nature of the care and support we provided would never have been realized.

4. Stewart Scharfman, MS, PT. When confronted with patients who continued to hurt, as a result of sore and fatigued muscles, it was Stewart who had the hands and the personality to lower the temperature, reduce the pain, and provide the emotional support over the course of treatment.

5. Fran Wolfe, chief librarian for the American Dental Association headquarters in Chicago. Her enthusiasm for our project and her ability to search out information enabled us to put in place all of the goals we had set out. Without her support this book could never have been written

6. John Bonica, MD. In my eyes, he is one of the key players who started the search for the tools to manage chronic, benign pain. His pains in the knees and hips, a result of intercollegiate wrestling, prompted his efforts to form the International Association for the Study of Pain (IASP). I was one of the charter members who met in Seattle in 1973.

## Special Thanks

As we tried to identify all of those who made it possible to write this book, the one who stands out is Debby Young. Before one word was put on paper and before our ideas were fully fleshed out, it was Debby who brought her skills to the table as a talented editor, writer and project manager. Though initially unfamiliar with the topic of facial pain, her insights and research were critical in defining the focus and personal perspectives that would be shared in this book. Of even more importance was her capacity to be exceedingly patient, supportive and critical, as we worked to stitch together viewpoints that sometimes diverged, as a result of our professional experiences that were defined by different times. Finding solutions, however, to the challenges that arose was her unique skill. Ultimately she functioned as a colleague, advisor, and confidant through the creation of this book. We are grateful for her effort.

# CONTENTS

# FOREWORD

Jeffrey P. Okeson, DMD

Professor and Chair, Department of Oral Health Science, Provost's Distinguished
Professorship, Director, Orofacial Pain Program, University of Kentucky College of Dentistry

Pain is the most powerful negative emotion that humans experience. It demands attention and response. Acute pain alarms the individual to the injury, which allows the sufferer to address the threat. Acute pain provides protection from environmental challenges. It is basic to survival and, therefore, has purpose. Some pains, however, last far longer than normal healing time and, therefore, have little protective value. These pains are termed chronic. They can become destructive to the human spirit, and lead to significant reduction in the quality of life. Some of the most common types of chronic pains originate from musculoskeletal structures. Chronic back, neck, and face pain are very frequent in the general population. These pains are typically dull, achy pains that can significantly decrease the individual's ability to function. This loss of function further compromises the quality of the individual's life.

Not only does chronic pain devastate individual sufferers emotionally, but its economic impact on society is enormous. In the United States alone, billions of dollars are spent each year on pain management.

Chronic pain in the limbs and back certainly impacts the quality of life to a great extent, yet for patients suffering with chronic facial pain, additional emotional elements become important considerations. It is interesting to note that approximately 45% of the human sensory cortex is dedicated to the face, mouth and oral structures. This degree of sensory dedication suggests that these structures have significant meaning to the individual, especially as regards pain. For example, pain in the orofacial structures significantly limits the individual's ability to chew, which is, of course, essential for survival. Although in these modern times we can sustain life without chewing (e.g., through the use of liquid diets, stomach tubes and intravenous feeding), we instinctively know that the inability to feed threatens one's existence. Therefore, chronic pain in the face threatens one's survival. Also, pain in the orofacial structures compromises the ability to speak, which is essential in a society dependent upon communication. In addition, chronic orofacial pain jeopardizes the individual's ability to successfully engage in society both at work and at play.

Another aspect of chronic orofacial pain that often goes unrecognized is the emotional component. The orofacial structures are very important to the individual for the expression of one's emotions. The smiles and frowns, the laughter and the tears are all expressed by our faces. Intimate activities such as kissing are also compromised by pain in the face. Therefore, one might appreciate that pain felt in the orofacial structures is much more threatening, meaningful and personal than pain felt in other areas of the body. Patients and doctors need to understand and appreciate that these psychologic factors accompany orofacial pain, especially as the pain becomes chronic.

A very important part in managing facial pain is to understand its origin. Often if the patient knows the cause and the natural course of the disorder, he or she can significantly influence the pain condition. This, of course, begins with education and is the rationale for this book. Drs. Tanenbaum and Roistacher have done an excellent job of accumulating a wealth of information for the pain patient to understand and appreciate. This book provides information that will assist patients in managing many different pain conditions. It is a valuable tool for improving the quality of life. Of course, pain conditions need to be initially assessed by qualified healthcare providers, but once this has been accomplished, this book can be very powerful in reducing the patient's suffering. Some of the guidelines given may seem simple, but we have learned that they are very powerful. I believe this book will be a very helpful tool for many pain sufferers. It will allow the patient to actively participate in his or her pain management. This is often essential for success. I highly recommend this book to all pain sufferers.

# INTRODUCTION

*The greatest mistake in the treatment of diseases is that there are physicians for the body and physicians for the soul, although the two cannot be separated.* — Plato

According to several independent studies, the annual incidence of people who experience facial pain is about 25% of the population (Goulet, Lavigne & Lund, 1995; McMillan, Wong, & Zheng, 2006). In America, that percentage equals about 75 million people. For many, pain is short-lived, particularly when associated with a tooth or sinus problem that is easy to recognize and predictably treated. Others, however, are less fortunate, as their suffering continues despite ongoing treatments that are recommended to address the site(s) of their reported pain. For this group of patients who often see internists, neurologists, otolaryngologists and multiple dental practitioners based on symptom location, pain lingers because ongoing investigations continue to search for disease or injury when, in fact, neither is present. As a result of this misdirected focus, the true origin of their pains, tense muscles of the face, jaw and neck, are overlooked.

While these specific muscle pain problems impact millions of people (4-12% of the U. S. population), they have drawn limited attention from the dental and medical communities. Medical records from our offices dating back to the early 1960s, which depict the wandering of facial pain patients as they searched for answers, unfortunately resemble the laments of today's patients who, after being shuttled from office to office, have been told, "There is nothing wrong" or "Live with your pain." Other patients have assuredly been told that they have migraines or neuralgia when, in fact, neither of these diagnoses were accurate. At a time of ad-vances in science and technology, why have these problems remained such a mystery and what needs to be done to change the perceptions of health-care providers confronted with these problems?

As dentists who have specialized in the study and treatment of oro-facial pain for several decades, we have come to understand the nature

1

of this most common expression of facial pain (driven by tense muscles) and how to alleviate it. Our understanding is based on a combined practice experience of nearly 70 years, spanning the past 4 decades, successfully treating thousands of patients suffering from severe and often persistent facial pain and related symptoms. Our understanding is also based on our participation and leadership roles in professional organizations devoted to the study and treatment of pain, including the American Pain Society (of which Dr. Roistacher was a founding member) and the American Academy of Orofacial Pain (of which Dr. Tanenbaum is a past president).

Despite our specialized training in pain management and experience as practitioners, we continue to be perplexed by the fact that very few people know what an "orofacial pain doctor" is, what we do, or—when all else has failed—how to locate a "facial pain doctor"—the phrase we will use from this point on to describe our specialty. Limited awareness of facial pain doctors exists even among most dentists and physicians, despite the existence of the American Academy of Orofacial Pain, which has many member-practitioners, and other organizations devoted to the study and treatment of facial pain.

Due to limited awareness and knowledge, most patients with lingering facial pain are left suffering, perplexed, and depressed when their pain cannot be properly diagnosed or treated by dentists or physicians, such as neurologists, allergists, or otolaryngologists (ear, nose, and throat doctors); and these doctors do not know where to refer patients whom they are unable to effectively help. As a result, millions of patients annually either suffer needlessly or are put through the diagnostic and treatment "mill" unnecessarily.

Although there are many books about headaches and TMJ (temporomandibular joint) disorders, for both the lay reader and healthcare professional, none of them focus exclusively on the recognition and treatment of the most common source of chronic facial pain problems, the muscles. That is why we wrote this book—to fill the void in the literature, with the hope of helping both lay readers and interested professionals to diagnose and effectively treat these problems in the least costly, time-consuming and stressful way possible.

Long before we envisioned writing this book, however, pioneers in the field of chronic pain, such as John Bonica, MD, who wrote the influential work *The Management of Pain* (1953), were also struggling to find answers for patients suffering as a result of unsolved causes of their pain. In their wisdom, clinicians like Bonica and fellow researchers formed the International Association for the Study of Pain (IASP) to facilitate the sharing of knowledge among healthcare practitioners.

Over the next several decades, various physicians began to lay the foundation for understanding how tense muscles, rather than structural, neurological, or other physical factors, could give rise to elusive and often debilitating pain symptoms. John Sarno, MD, was especially influential in this regard, with his revolutionary book *Mind Over Back Pain* (1984).

As a result of the knowledge we gained from the pioneers in pain research, and our professional training and experience, it became evident that most of our facial pain patients were in trouble despite the absence of disease or classic tissue injury. Our search for answers, therefore, could not focus only on specific physical causes. Rather, if we were to help these patients, we would need to identify other factors, which we eventually concluded were emotional—and could comprise the brain's ability to keep muscles comfortable.

As the years passed, we concluded that there was a need for this book.

## An Overview of the General Perspective of this Book

Medical researchers and theorists have explored the intimate connection between the mind and the body for years, in the quest to understand illnesses associated with the heart, skin, back, and gastrointestinal system, but this book is the first to apply the mind-body model to facial pain. By focusing on the relationship between emotions and muscles, we uncover the mystery of seemingly "unsolvable" pain problems and provide answers to questions such as the following: Why would a person experience a persistent toothache despite the fact that the tooth that hurts is structurally sound? Why would a person gradually lose the ability to open his or her mouth or talk when no recognizable injury had occurred or medical disease been identified? Why would a person experience a relentless ache or pain in his or her face despite all medical evaluations suggesting that "there is nothing wrong?"

The reason muscles are such an important cause of facial pain is that the face is mainly composed of muscles, and muscles are second only to

3

the teeth in giving rise to facial pain problems. These facts are not commonly known by healthcare practitioners, which helps explain why so many of them overlook the role of muscles when confronted with patients complaining of facial pain.

Despite the chronic nature of patients' problems and suggestions by many practitioners that their symptoms are "in their head," our experience has clearly revealed that problematic reactions of the muscles of the jaw, other facial areas, and the neck occur as a result of emotions, and the impact of life-challenges on the brain. We call this state a brain "under siege." As explained in detail in this book, a brain under siege from negative emotions, inability to express anger, difficult life circumstances, loss of control in one's daily life, or the relentless pursuit of achievement often leads to neural and physical changes expressed as muscle pain in the face and neck.

This explanation is more vital to understand than ever before in our history, because we are living through an unprecedented number of challenges that stand in the way of the pursuit of happiness and emotional contentment. Americans are experiencing higher levels of stress, it may be argued, brought on by factors such as the persistent economic recession, a divorce rate hovering around 50%, unemployment reaching levels not seen since the Great Depression, the obligation of Baby Boomers to take care of aging parents with Alzheimer's disease or other medical infirmities, and the loss of the extended family as an unfaltering last line of support. This society-wide condition largely explains why the number of people experiencing facial pain, driven by fatigued and dysfunctional muscles, has significantly increased.

In relating the brain and emotions to facial pain, we realize that you—like the majority of people—may be tempted to reject this explanatory model. The reason this model (or theory) is so strongly rejected in our Western culture is that we have grown up believing in the "duality" of the mind and the body, and thus tend to automatically look for structural, neurological, or other material causes of pain in almost all instances. As a result, we discount mental or emotional factors as responsible for physical pain-related symptoms. This skeptical reaction exists even among the great majority of healthcare professionals. Although the biological mechanisms by which emotions prompt the onset of muscle tension and facial pain are well understood by those involved in research, dental and medical practitioners involved in patient care are either uncomfortable or ineffective in communicating this reality to their patients.

We want to emphasize that we are not implying that information about emotional factors alone is sufficient to alleviate many types of facial pain symptoms. Nor do we minimize the use of traditional pain-relieving approaches to symptom relief. In fact, in this book we describe the many types of physical treatments—from pain medications to muscle relaxants to oral appliances and physiotherapy—that we, and other facial pain doctors, provide for patients. Each patient, however, needs to be viewed as an individual, with his or her own symptoms and history, and treated accordingly.

Our overriding goal in this book is to make it clear that though almost all facial muscle pain problems are reversible, they require patient insight and participation during the process of feeling better. These problems are not, in short, "doctor, fix me" problems, but, rather, problems that are personal in origin and require personal attention and effort, if both short- and long-term symptom reduction is to be realized. We believe that a full understanding of what we share in this book will give sufferers the control they need to keep their muscles comfortable and thereby reduce or eliminate their facial pain.

It is our final hope, therefore, that this book will help ease patients' suffering and also inspire healthcare professionals to expand their horizons, as they try to meet the challenges of their profession. If we are successful in our mission, we will have taken an important step toward managing a problem that exacts a huge personal toll on millions of patients every year.

# Chapter 1

# DEFINING THE FACE AND FACIAL PAIN

*Was this the face that launch'd a thousand ships and burnt the topless towers of Ilium?*
— Christopher Marlowe, *Dr. Faustus*

In these lines about Helen of Troy, Marlowe poetically conveys the central place of the face in human life. Though few of us may have a "face that could launch a thousand ships," every person has the same face as Helen in the most essential respects: It is the front part of our head that goes from the forehead to the chin, and includes the sensory organs—nose, eyes, ears, and tongue—as well as the cheeks, lips, mouth, teeth, and jaw. Figure 1 below shows the boundaries of the face.

Figure 1: The Boundaries of the Face

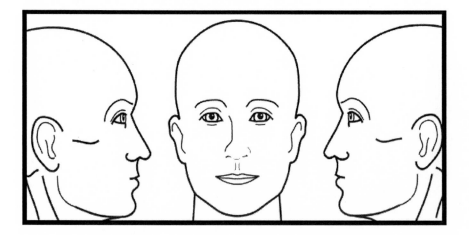

We also share with Helen the potential to experience pain in any part of the face, or *facial pain*. Under the broad umbrella of facial pain, there can be a multitude of pain problems that stem from the teeth, sinuses, ears, eyes, and oral soft tissues. Fortunately pain problems associated with these structures are often clear in their presentation, such as the common toothache, headache, or earache, and are managed well after accurate diagnosis. These problems, therefore, often don't become persistent and are not specifically those that we address in this book.

As facial pain doctors, we are mainly concerned with pain-related symptoms that occur in the sensory organs, the mouth and the jaw; but we also diagnose and treat symptoms in the scalp and the neck, the two areas contiguous with the face. The neck—which connects the head to the trunk of the body—is often of special interest to us, and sometimes even the shoulders, because they share nerves with the face that can be responsible for facial pain symptoms.

While each person is intimately familiar with how his or her face appears in the mirror, and is concerned about how others see it, few people realize that behind its external appearance the face is composed mainly of *muscles*. By using certain facial muscles we show emotions, such as sadness, happiness, confusion, surprise, and excitement, which enable us to communicate on a social level; and, of course, we use the mouth, jaw, teeth and tongue to speak, eat and swallow—vital functions that are controlled mainly by muscles.

Given the prominence of muscles in the facial area, the focus of this book is on facial pain of muscle origin, and the consequences that muscular compromise inflicts on the neural and vascular structures contained within muscles and their associated tendons. Knowing how to recognize the symptoms related to facial pain of muscular origin, therefore, and understanding what causes facial muscles to hurt are the keys to seeking proper treatment.

What are the symptoms of facial pain, especially those you should be most concerned about? Why do facial muscles hurt and what can be done to alleviate or eradicate the pain? What is the correct type of treatment for most types of persistent facial pain? These and related questions are answered in the following chapters of this book.

## Summary

The face is the visible, front part of the head that contains our sensory organs and the cheeks, mouth, teeth, lips, and jaw. While we all have the potential to experience pain in any part of the face, facial pain doctors are mainly concerned with symptoms that are persistent and often debilitating. The face is composed primarily of muscles, which are often the main source of facial pain. It is, therefore, important to know how to recognize the symptoms related to facial pain of muscular origin, and to understand what causes facial muscles to hurt. These are the keys to getting the proper treatment for most facial pain.

## Chapter 2

# THE SYMPTOMS AND PATTERNS OF FACIAL PAIN

*God hath given you one face, and you make yourselves another.* — Shakespeare, *Hamlet*

## The Variety of Facial Pain Symptoms and Presentations

Patients with facial pain report a wide variety of symptoms, which sometimes also include odd sensations and mobility problems. Many of the symptoms are commonplace and readily understandable while others are unusual and enigmatic. Among the variety of symptoms that facial pain patients report are the following: "My forehead is sore," "My jaw is tight," "The hair on my scalp is sensitive," "My ears ache," "My face is never relaxed," "I feel pins and needles in my face," "I can't bring my teeth together," "My ears are clogged," "I can't open my mouth fully," "I can't chew food," "My face feels numb," "My ears feel full," "My teeth ache," "My gums feel tight," "My face feels like someone punched me," "My jaw feels like it does not belong to me," "I feel spasms in my face," "My jaw feels misaligned," "My cheeks feel hot," and "I feel tingling in my face." Despite these symptoms, the physical appearance of many facial pain sufferers prompts doctors to say, "You look great, it is hard to believe that you hurt so much." The insinuation that their symptoms are not real troubles many of our patients.

In addition to these types of symptoms—which involve "feeling states" (of pain and/or odd sensations)—some patients also display signs of their suffering by a creased forehead, a braced jaw, clenched teeth, raised shoulders, forward head posture, and a shallow breathing tendency. As you will soon learn, people often exhibit such physical behaviors and postures when they are emotionally upset, and these factors further contribute to the generation and experience of facial pain.

9

## Three Categories of Common Symptoms

The symptoms that are described by patients with facial pain can be grouped into one of three categories: (1) symptoms that feature pain *per se* (sensory expression); (2) symptoms that feature altered sensations such as feelings of numbness or warmth in the facial region (neural expression); and (3) symptoms that feature muscle tension or contracture (motor expression).

Most facial pain patients with these symptoms initially seek relief from dentists and various types of medical specialists, such as an ENT (ear, nose and throat) doctor, an allergist, or a neurologist, before they see a facial pain doctor. This scenario—of people with confusing facial pain symptoms who seek initial professional consultation and unsuccessful treatment—is well illustrated by two of our patients, Sarah and Karen.

Sarah was a well-educated, intelligent, attractive woman, 43 years of age, when she first came for treatment. Though she had kind eyes and a warm smile, her sadness was apparent from her demeanor. She had been struggling with facial pain for over a year, especially jaw and tooth pain. On her first visit she tearfully reported that three of her teeth had been treated with root canal therapy, but her pain continued every day, accompanied by a pulling across her jaw muscles and a sense that she could not open her mouth fully. Sarah's symptoms also included severe scalp sensitivity and pain on the left side of her face, which interfered with ordinary activities. She couldn't put the left side of her face on her pillow, blow-dry her hair, or even kiss her husband without experiencing pain. Her whole world had become consumed by pain and she didn't know what to do or where to go. "You're my last hope," she said, revealing her frustration after having seen ear, nose, and throat specialists (who prescribed antibiotics), internists (who prescribed valium), and neurologists (who told her to take medications to ease the pain)—all to no avail. She could not recall a specific incident or event that had triggered her pain but, rather, the pain had come on gradually and had intensified over time. "Pain greets me in the morning and is the last thing I think about before I go to bed at night," Sarah said.

Another patient, Karen, was 37 years old when she came for treatment. She was accompanied by her husband, who had little patience for this consultation after seeing a long line of doctors. Though Karen was obviously in pain, she was most concerned about the odd sensations in her face. She described numbness and tingling in her jaw and other facial areas, and she was concerned that her face felt lopsided and swollen. Karen also mentioned that she felt her teeth were not touching properly and her jaw muscles felt fatigued. When her husband was asked about the doctors she had already seen, he answered, "She has seen more doctors in the last 6 months than I have seen in my lifetime. They all think that whatever she is feeling is in her head."

## Multiple Symptoms and Locations

As you've just seen in the cases of Sarah and Karen, facial pain patients can experience a variety of symptoms simultaneously in different parts of the facial area, or even in the scalp, neck, and shoulders. Patients with pain *per se* in the ears (sensory expression), for example, may also experience numbness (neural expression) in the cheeks; patients with tight jaw muscles (motor expression) may also experience a burning sensation in the forehead (neural expression); patients with tingling in the scalp (neural expression) may also experience tension in the neck (motor expression) and pain in the jaw (sensory expression). As you can surmise from these examples and the foregoing discussion, there are a great many symptoms reported by this patient population, and an even greater number of ways the symptoms can combine in any given individual.

## Patterns of Facial Pain Symptoms

The many different types of symptoms associated with facial pain are often ephemeral and exhibit many varied patterns. Facial pain symptoms, for example, can be sharp or dull, come on suddenly or slowly emerge, last a short while or a long time, or be localized or "spread out."

When people experience symptoms that are longstanding, intense, or puzzling, such as a tingling sensation that emerges in the cheeks and spreads in a seemingly random, unpredictable pattern to their lips and tongue, they often become frightened, and sink into a state of hopelessness and despair.

While facial pain in the population that we see usually comes on gradually, some people experience the onset of pain suddenly. You could be completely pain free one day and in severe pain the next, without any awareness of why this has happened. Symptoms might come on during a common physical event like yawning, eating or smiling, or you might not be able to identify a specific triggering action. Either way, when people experience an abrupt onset of pain, they usually believe they have suffered an injury. As you will see, however, this belief is usually unfounded, because nothing injurious has happened to the face.

With facial pain, the severity of symptoms can vary considerably from moment to moment or day to day—a pattern that differs from, say, pain that arises from physical injuries you may have sustained in the past. It is not uncommon for our patients to tell us that some days they can eat a bagel sandwich without any problems and then 2 days later experience sharp jaw pain when they eat a bowl of pasta. Other patients report that on some days their face hurts just by smiling.

When this cycle continues to repeat itself, it becomes clear to us that the specific action, such as chewing or smiling, is only a trigger; and the focus of attention, therefore, needs to be on the condition of the jaw or other facial muscles long before the triggering action occurs. On days when eating soft food gives rise to intense pain, for example, it is more than likely that the jaw muscles entered into the chewing process already fatigued and incapable of sustaining normal function.

## Referred Pain

If you went to the town doctor 100 years ago complaining of left arm pain, treatment would have focused on the left arm and the associated muscles, tendons, ligaments, and bones. At that time in medical history, the understanding of pain was dominated by the teaching of the philosopher René Descartes, who theorized that pain was experienced as a result of a nerve being noxiously stimulated in one part of the body. As a result, signals were sent directly to the brain where perception of this painful body part occurred. (Descartes is most famous, perhaps, for arguing that the "mind" and "body" are inherently separate. We disagree strongly with this viewpoint and explain why in Chapter 5, along with important implications for facial pain patients.)

Today we have come a long way from Descartes' simple understanding of pain transmission. We now know that, at times, the location of pain has little to do with the source of the pain. When the source of your pain is not the body part that actually hurts, the pain is called *referred* pain. We now understand, for example, that left arm pain may have nothing to do with the arm, but may be the first warning sign of an impending heart attack. In the same way, when patients have facial pain, such as in the jaw, teeth, or ear, there may be nothing wrong with those structures, because the pain is being referred from elsewhere in the facial area or possibly even from the neck or shoulders.

In fact, referred pain and associated muscle tightening can occur in unpredictable ways, producing symptoms that vary in intensity, frequency, and duration. When referral mechanisms are responsible for pain symptoms, medical and dental examinations often produce little information, and patients leave doctors' offices often more confused and anxious than they were prior to the consultation.

Referred facial pain is one of the key reasons dentists and medical specialists often misdiagnose facial pain, and why their treatments fail to bring relief to their patients. (See Chapter 4 for a full discussion of why dentists and physicians often misunderstand and misdiagnose facial pain.)

## *Trigger Points and Referred Pain*

Based on the teachings of Hans Kraus (1965) and others (Simons, Simons, & Travel, 1983), we have come to appreciate that pain in the facial area—including the teeth, lips, ears, eyes, forehead, nose, and sinuses—may be present as a result of highly sensitive sources of pain in the muscles of the jaw, neck, and even the shoulders. These sources of referred pain are called *trigger points*, and when they are stimulated, pain is felt in a distant location. The referred pain that results is usually dull and aching, and is increased as the trigger points are stimulated by repeated muscle contractions.

Research has shown that there is an intimate relationship between nerve pathways in the jaw and other facial areas and those in the cervical spine, i.e., the upper part of the spine in the neck region (Simons, Simons, & Travel, 1983). In addition, pain is most commonly referred towards the head. As a result, it is extremely common for muscles in the neck and shoulder region to refer pain to the jaw and other facial areas. Many of our patients over the years have come to us with a variety of symptoms that have not responded to treatment focused only on the location of the symptoms. We have treated these patients successfully, however, by identifying the source of the pain symptoms as muscles of the neck and shoulders. These sources of referred pain are shown in Figures 2A and

2B, where "x" represents the origin of the pain and the dotted areas ("targets") represent where the pain is felt.

Figure 2A: Referred Pain to the Face and Jaw from the Sternocleidomastoid Muscles

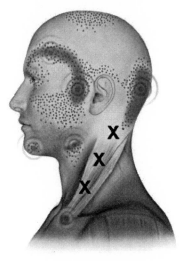

Figure 2B: Referred Pain to the Face and Jaw from the Trapezius Muscles

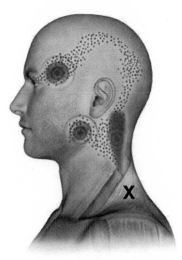

## The Jaw and Referred Pain

The jaw muscles, as mentioned, also have the capacity to trigger pain symptoms in other facial areas. The ears, teeth, sinus, and back of the eye, for example, are just a few of the common locations where people experience pain as a result of referral from the muscles that open and close your mouth and move your jaw from side to side or forward and back. These symptoms are quite common when the jaw is in use, but may also occur spontaneously when the jaw is at rest. These sources of referred pain are shown in Figures 3A and 3B, where "x" represents the origin of the pain and the dotted areas ("targets") represent where the pain is felt.

Figure 3A: Referred Pain to the Teeth, Ear, Sinus and
Face from the Masseter Muscle

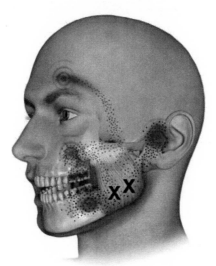

Figure 3B: Referred Pain to the Teeth, Ear, Sinus and
Face from the Temporalis Muscle

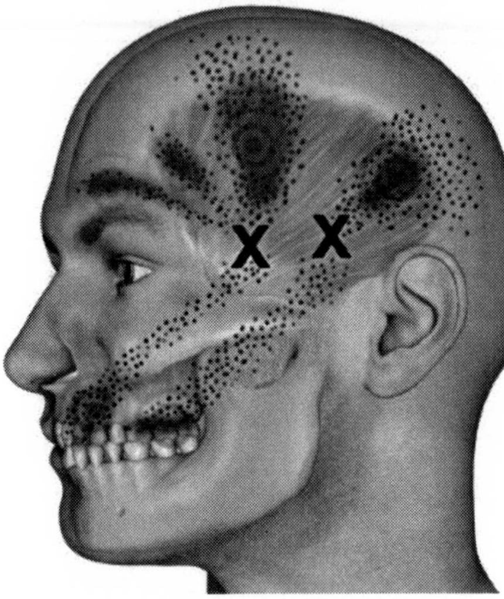

## Recurring Pain

Though the vast majority of patients who have experienced facial pain as a result of muscles can experience relief, pain symptoms may recur, or re-emerge, often with no predictable pattern or for any readily identifiable reasons. This is especially so if the patient's pain is related to stressful life conditions, as you'll see in some of the case histories we present later in the book. As a result, a chronic cycle of pain and discomfort impacts our patients not only during their normal, daily routine, but even when they are trying to relax, such as on a vacation. These patients may be ready to feel well, but their muscles are so overworked and fatigued that they are limited in their capacity to recover. With an inability to feel better even when removed from their stressful work or home environments, these patients are inclined to continually embrace the concept that there must be injury or medical disease driving their symptoms. Other patients tell us they feel well during vacation, but when they get back to home and work obligations, the symptoms re-emerge. For these patients, it is easy to accept a connection between their emotional state and re-emergent muscle pain symptoms.

16

## Fluctuating Pain

Fluctuation in symptom intensity is another pattern that exists among many facial pain patients. Their suffering, for example, may be extreme at certain times during the same day while at other times it can be at a much lower level. This pattern of pain variability is often very disruptive to patients' lives, since they cannot predict when they will get into trouble again and, therefore, they have a hard time planning social and work-related activities.

## Sleep and Facial Pain Symptoms

In the context of this discussion, it is important to note the relationship between facial pain symptoms and sleep. While emotions and learned behaviors can seemingly cause or increase symptoms related to facial muscle pain, especially "empty" behaviors such as clenching the teeth and bracing the jaw muscles (see Chapter 5 for a detailed discussion of this relationship), the quantity and quality of sleep we get also appears to be a significant factor that affects the nature and intensity of facial pain symptoms (Lavigne et al., 2007).

As we all know, insufficient sleep has become epidemic in our society. The many factors that typically impact sleep include general anxiety about health, job security, income, and marriage and family issues. In addition, concern about ongoing medical conditions; persistent pain problems, such as those in the neck and back; drinking caffeine or alcohol prior to bedtime; shift work; and medications like antidepressants, decongestants, and sleeping pills that have been used over an extended period of time also impact the quality and quantity of sleep.

To understand the relationship between sleep and pain in general, consider what happens when you are deprived of sleep, both in terms of quantity and quality. Research has shown that after a few days of sleep deprivation the body begins to shut down—body temperature regulation is lost, blood pressure fluctuates, immune systems are damaged, mood and memory capacity are altered, cellular mechanisms for growth and repair are compromised, and muscle and joint pain emerge throughout the body. In addition, research by Michael Smith (2004), at Johns Hopkins University, suggests that when sleep is disturbed the body's natural pain inhibitory functions are profoundly impaired. This condition leads to spontaneous pain symptoms.

These findings strongly suggest that the relationship between disturbed sleep and pain is bi-directional, meaning not only does pain disrupt sleep, but the reverse is also true, i.e., disrupted sleep likely exacerbates pain, and can lead to pain in the absence of a specific event or set of easily identifiable contributing factors.

## Summary

There are many types of facial pain symptoms, which can exist alone or in combination. Most of them involve "feeling states," such as pain (sensory expression) or odd sensations (neural expression), while others involve muscle tension or contracture (motor expression). Facial pain symptoms can affect any specific part of the face or exist in multiple locations at the same time.

In addition to their great variety, facial pain symptoms exhibit various types of patterns. They can be sharp or dull, come on suddenly or slowly emerge, last a short while or a long time, be acute or chronic, or be localized or "spread out," among other patterns. The symptoms can appear during a common event, like yawning or eating, or for no apparent reason at all. The severity of symptoms also can vary considerably from moment to moment or day to day. Facial pain that is felt in a specific location, such as the eyes or ears, may be referred from the neck or the jaw. As a result of referred pain symptoms, there is often misdiagnosis and ineffective treatment. While emotions and learned or "empty" behaviors can cause or exacerbate facial pain symptoms, the quantity and quality of sleep we get also appears to be a significant risk factor that affects the nature and intensity of common facial pain symptoms.

# Chapter 3

# WHO HAS PERSISTENT FACIAL PAIN?

*It is much more important to know what sort of patient has a disease than what sort of disease a patient has.* — Sir William Osler

Everyone has pain in the facial area at some point in life, especially if we consider commonplace toothaches and headaches. In addition, most people have an earache, a "stiff neck," or a sore jaw at one time or another, among other rather common sources of facial pain and discomfort. While such types of pain are often short-lived and transient, many individuals at any given time have more serious or chronic problems involving facial pain. Who are the millions of Americans who experience persistent facial pain each year? The answer to this question will probably surprise you.

## Characteristics of Facial Pain Patients

Overall, the great majority of facial pain patients are between the ages of 20 and 50, with an average age of 34, and about 80% of them are women (Jensen et al., 1993). This gender difference among facial pain patients is seemingly enigmatic, but it may be explained by several different types of factors that differentiate men and women, which are discussed shortly in this chapter.

A focused assessment of this population of patients whom we have routinely seen reveals that they are immersed in the years of responsibility. They are taking care of or trying to conceive children, working hard to pay the bills and succeed in life, aspiring to attain goals they have set, and beginning to assume the role of providing care to ill or aging parents. They are the youngest of the "sandwich generation," trying to make ends meet while at the same time living up to their own and society's expectations. In addition it is our impression that most of our patients either had great

19

stress in their lives at the time of their visits or they had experienced persistent emotional upset or loss of control—often related to family, work, health, money, security, or some other important aspect of their lives. This critical connection—between people's experience of facial pain and emotional upset—is discussed in detail in subsequent chapters of the book (see Chapter 5, especially, for a full explanation of the link between a brain "under siege" and facial muscle pain).

Along with the most commonly seen group of patients (20-50 years of age) we also see teenagers and seniors of both sexes, whose numbers have been increasing over the last decade or so. We believe this is also likely due to the increased number and severity of "stressors" in society that are affecting the emotional lives of all people, even teenagers, as may be seen in the case of 15-year-old Emily.

Emily was upbeat and did not appear to be in pain as she walked into the office with both of her parents. Despite experiencing facial pain for a year and a half, she smiled as she chatted about her life as a high school sophomore. When asked to rate her level of pain on a scale from 1-10, with 10 being the most severe, she said, "I hurt all the time and my pain is a 10 every day." She felt pain in her face and ear, and had headaches in her temples on a daily basis. In addition, Emily's jaw muscles felt sore and tired and she had longstanding tension in her neck and upper back. She had seen a neurologist, an oral surgeon, and her pediatrician prior to coming to our office, but none of these doctors could offer a specific diagnosis. Like most of our patients with facial pain, Emily could not identify a traumatic event or medical problem that triggered the pain.

As Emily continued to talk, it was noticed that she continually held her lower lip between her teeth and braced her jaw forward. As a result, one could see the tension she held in her face. When asked how many hours she slept, Emily estimated 6 hours a night, which prompted a look of great concern on her parents' faces. "I can't sleep more. I'm too busy with school," Emily said, obviously annoyed at the implication that she needed more sleep. When she was asked, "Are you an A student and involved in lots of clubs and extracurricular activities?" she remarked, "Why should you care about that? I came here so you could get rid of my pain."

With these facts in place—especially the lack of any identifiable physical, structural, or neurological problem—it appeared that Emily's focus on school achievement at the expense of adequate sleep and relaxation had likely triggered her pain symptoms.

## Why Are Most Facial Pain Patients Women?

As mentioned above, most facial pain patients are women. Whether the diagnosis is muscle pain, temporomandibular dysfunction (TMD), or a tension headache, women fill our schedules on a daily basis. What could explain this difference between the sexes in the facial pain patient population? In attempting to answer this question, there appear to be a number of factors that significantly differentiate men and women when it comes to facial pain.

### Gender-Specific Differences and Facial Pain

Experts in gender-specific medicine, such as Marianne Legato, MD, at Columbia University in New York City, believe men and women are significantly different in the way they experience illness (Legato, 2008). These differences are likely due to a combination of biological, psychological, and social factors—including hormones, genetics, cognitive and emotional processes, and the effects of imposed stereotypical roles. Research studies that have examined the experience of facial muscle pain have revealed that women experience symptoms at an earlier age than men and that their pain lasts longer than that of men (Fillingim et al., 2005). In addition, contrary to common beliefs, the dominance of women in facial pain practices is not mainly due to care seeking behaviors (Macfarlane, 2003) but is rather due to the severity of their pain symptoms (Levitt & McKinney, 1994).

Other investigators have identified several physiological factors that predispose women to musculoskeletal problems and facial pain. Recent research at the University of Michigan, for example, suggests that differences between men and women in the perception and experience of sustained pain can be due in part to the influence of gonadal hormones (estrogen) on the brain (Cahill & Akil, 2006). Cyclic fluctuations in estrogen have, in fact, been associated with the activation of various factors that influence inflammation, pain threshold and pain perception (Aloisi & Bonifazi, 2006). A role of gonadal hormones in pain mechanisms is also supported by data showing the effects of exogenous hormones (hormone replacement therapy, oral contraceptives) on intensifying the pain experience (LeResche et al., 1997). Differences in the structural organization and function of the sympathetic nervous system (the part of the nervous system responsible for the fight or flight response) may also partially explain gender differences in pain.

In addition, from a biological perspective, female jaw muscles have less endurance than their male counterparts. This is due to less capillary density in the jaw muscles of females, which means less blood flow. In general, less blood flow will bring less oxygen, predisposing the jaw muscles to quicker fatigue and associated soreness and pain.

While a consensus has not been reached to explain this great disparity between the number of men and women who seek care for common facial pain problems, it is likely that biological differences play a critical role.

## The Expression of Anger

Men and women express anger differently (Dittmann, 2003). This behavioral disparity, which begins in childhood (Chaplin, Cole & Zahn-Waxler, 2005), is important to consider when trying to understand the preponderance of women with facial pain. For men, anger is often expressed the instant a conflict arises, whether it is in the home or workplace. The response may be verbal, physical, or both, but the outcome is the same: men tend to quickly "blow off steam." A vivid example is the common response of a major league baseball manager who considers an umpire's call to be unfair and to the detriment of his team. He comes charging out of the dugout, gets in the umpire's face, and screams and kicks dirt as his own face and ears turn bright red. Within moments the confrontation is over, the manager is thrown out of the game and retreats to the clubhouse, where he is likely to be congratulated for his efforts to inspire his team. Not only has he successfully released his anger and frustration (which may well have been building up due to his team's poor performance), but he has also gained the respect of his players for standing up for the team. He is, for the moment, actually a hero!

For women, however, this overt and public display of anger generally would be considered unacceptable. Women are usually more contemplative and less spontaneous than men in their response to conflict, and their display of anger is often muted or not revealed at all. As a consequence, we believe that women often pay a price physically, with the end result being pain in the muscles of the face and neck. Whether ongoing conflicts at home or work drive learned behaviors (such as braced jaw muscles and clenched teeth) or activate the autonomic nervous system (which controls such things as muscle tone, blood circulation, nerve discharge and heart rate), the stage is set for symptoms to develop over time.

Most recently one of our patients said, "I have been a people pleaser for my entire life, but I am at the end of my rope, particularly at work. My boss throws balls in the air all day long and expects me to catch them, no matter what else I have to accomplish. I have had enough, but I can't replace this job or the health benefits. It really gets you after a while."

In our experience, therefore, buried feelings and emotions that have no outlet or can't be expressed for fear of negative consequences (such as physical or verbal assault from a spouse or boyfriend, divorce, or loss of a job) are a predictable reason why many of our women patients are in pain. The pain has a physical basis—muscle dysfunction (described in detail shortly below)—but the origin is deep-seated in buried emotions. When we review the emotional landscapes of many of our women patients, we often see personal conflicts and life challenges that have no easy answers. These factors must certainly be recognized and addressed if the strategies for pain relief we offer are to be successful over the long term.

### Help-Seeking Behavior and Facial Pain

As we work towards better understanding the patient with facial pain, it is also important to keep in mind that pain is an individual experience, with both a sensory component (sensation of pain) and a reactive component (seeking care). For all medical problems, women go to doctors eight or nine times more often than men do, and doctors tend to assign a diagnosis to women's complaints more frequently than they do for men. In addition, women in many societies are taught during childhood that seeking care for pain will not carry with it a lasting stigma of weakness. This is often contrary to the way men learn to respond to pain (Galdas, Cheater, & Marshall, 2005; Pilkey, 2011). To their credit, women tend to seek care early during their suffering, allowing for effective treatment strategies to be put into place. Some of our biggest challenges arise when a man seeks care long after his pain symptoms have first emerged.

## *Sleep, Women and Facial Pain*

A final factor to consider about sex differences and facial-related pain is the relationship between sleep and pain, as discussed at the end of Chapter 2. Some of the women we commonly see begin to experience facial pain when their sleep has been altered by the presence of a newborn. Many of them had been sound sleepers for years before giving birth, but they began to experience facial pain symptoms of significant magnitude for the first time when their sleep was continually disturbed by the newborn. In addition, they report that the use of over-the-counter medications for their pain is not helpful. This is not surprising, as research has shown that sleep deprivation and disruption can counter the benefits of pain medications.

## Social-Psychological Characteristics of Facial Pain Patients

In addition to their sex and age characteristics, many facial pain patients seem more likely than others to exhibit certain social and psychological characteristics. Some of these characteristics were first described by the American Pain Society, which referred to them as "the four faces of pain." These patients may be briefly described as follows:

1.    They are unable to make a connection between emotions and the presence of pain.

2.    They reject personal relationships in order to avoid social and emotional pain and distress.

3.    They ignore their own physical and emotional needs in order to take care of everyone else, while denying that their pain might be the result of this self-neglect.

4.    They withdraw from social contacts that provide support, distraction, and the other rewards of friendship.

While all of these social-psychological descriptions do not apply to every patient we have seen over the years, the first one listed—an inability to make a connection between emotions and the presence of pain—is common to the majority of our patients. We believe that the main reason for their lack of insight relates directly to the subtle and poorly understood mechanisms responsible for the emergence of muscle pain symptoms.

## Pain as a Symptom without Disease

As will be discussed at length in the chapters that follow, the pain experienced by the vast majority of facial pain patients is not the result of a structural problem, disease, illness, or injury. In fact, a large percentage of all facial pain arises in the absence of traumatic injury or disease. This, however, does not mean that the pain being experienced is any less real than pain that is caused by a specific event or disease. By definition, pain is the *perception by the brain* of an unpleasant sensation that is due to actual or potential tissue damage. It is a function of how the brain receives, interprets, and responds to nerve signals. Whether the nerve signals arrive at the brain as a result of a trauma, an aggressive disease process, or a persistently contracted and sore muscle, the brain's response and the experience of pain are essentially the same.

The critical concept that "there is no pain without the brain" makes it clear that the pain experience is not only based on the source of the pain signal but, most importantly, on the *interpretation* of the signal by the brain. If a person does not understand why he or she has pain, is fearful that the pain will not go away, or is anxious and overwhelmed by difficult life circumstances, then the sensation of pain will be heightened.

In order, then, to begin to understand how the most common facial pain (which is due to muscle) can develop without injury or disease, it is important to introduce the concept of "sensitization." Think of the sensitization process as the reason why you hurt after getting a sunburn. Your skin is more sensitive after a sunburn because the nerve endings in your skin have been irritated by the thermal energy of the sun. As a result, when you touch skin that is sunburned, it hurts. In fact, all normal stimuli applied to the skin, such as the fabric of a shirt or the water from a shower, is interpreted as pain. Similarly, the nerve endings in your muscles can be sensitized due to a change in the chemical environment in muscle tissue. These chemical changes occur in the presence of persistently contracted and tense muscles that are in trouble as a result of emotional turmoil and difficult life circumstances. Once sensitized, the threshold for nerves to fire in response to stimuli is lowered. In other words, once irritated, sensitized nerve endings will respond even to normal activities such as chewing or speaking. The pain that results from the stimulation of nerves with lowered thresholds will not go away until the source of irritation is removed.

As a result of sensitization, muscle pain emerges and, more importantly, is experienced long after one would have expected healing to occur. If patients do not suspect that their brain is involved in their pain, then the key source of continual irritation remains and symptoms continue. As a result, for many of our patients what started out as a localized pain evolves into a more widespread pain experience. Ultimately some of our patients not only hurt but they suffer, to the extent they have lost belief in the possibility of relief.

## There Is No Pill for Suffering

Pain and suffering are uniquely different, and it is important to understand the distinction. You can take a pill to relieve physical pain, since it is experienced by the body, but suffering is experienced by the mind and is more complex. Patients report high levels of suffering when the source of their pain is unknown and there is no identifiable cause. When you don't understand this situation, it can feel threatening, especially when a specific physical cause can't be identified. Unfortunately, when you feel that doctors judge your pain as "psychological" and, in a sense, not "real," you can lose confidence in the healthcare system, get very frustrated, and experience prolonged continuation of your pain. As you will see in some of the patient scenarios we describe in this book, it would have been far better if, somewhere along the line, some healthcare professional had said, "I don't know what is wrong with you but your symptoms are real." This simple statement would not only have represented the truth, but also created optimism that solutions were possible.

## Summary

At some point in life virtually everyone has a rather transient type of facial pain, such as a common toothache or headache, which is readily identifiable and treatable. If we ignore these common sources of facial pain, however, it is estimated that about 4-12% of the population has facial pain of muscle origin that is often persistent and confusing in its presentation (Goulet et al., 1995; Macfarlane et al., 2002; Nilsson et al., 2002). In terms of age and sex, most facial pain patients are middle age and women, with about 20% being men, teenagers and seniors. Over the past few decades, the number of both younger and older patients has been increasing, probably because of the greater number of stressors in society related to achievement, work, income, family responsibilities, and health.

While we cannot definitively say why most facial pain patients are women, the disparity in the sex ratio could be accounted for by gender-specific differences related to biology, psychology, and social factors; help-seeking behaviors related to socialization and cultural factors; and sleep patterns related to childbearing and caretaking.

In addition to their demographic characteristics, most facial pain patients appear to have certain social-psychological characteristics in common. Their case histories indicate that they are either undergoing a lot of stress at the time of treatment or have recently experienced great stress, and are in a state of emotional upset—a phenomenon we refer to as having a brain "under siege." In addition, many pain patients have one or more of the following characteristics, which the American Pain Society described as the "four faces of pain": They are unable to make a connection between emotions and the presence of pain; they reject personal relationships in order to avoid social and emotional pain and distress; they ignore their own needs and instead care for others while failing to recognize that their pain might be due to self-neglect; and they withdraw from friendly, supportive social relationships which could be a source of support.

## Chapter 4

## HOW MOST PATIENTS FIRST RESPOND TO PERSISTENT FACIAL PAIN — AND WHY THEY USUALLY FAIL TO GET RELIEF

*It is easy to get a thousand prescriptions but hard to get one single remedy.* — Chinese Proverb

If you are like most of our patients, you had facial pain that increased gradually over time, your symptoms were present for months or even years, and your pain eventually became unmanageable. When over-the-counter medications no longer worked sufficiently, you decided to see a dentist or physician, such as a neurologist or an ENT doctor. Failing to get a solution to your problem, you decided to go to a facial pain doctor on your own or were referred to one, most likely by your physician or dentist.

This frustrating process is clearly illustrated by the case of Jane, who describes what happened to her in her own words: "My pain started in-between two of my upper left molars. I was very scared because only a couple of months ago, I had just finished going through the traumatic experience of having a failed root canal on the other side of my mouth, followed by the extraction of the tooth. Prior to these episodes, I had been the easiest dental patient for over 30 years. I had two fillings in my mouth and basically went to the dentist only for check-ups. I couldn't help but wonder what on earth was going on with my mouth.

"Over the next month, I saw my dentist multiple times, an endodontist twice, and a periodontist, but no one could figure out the source of the pain. While I was going from dentist to dentist, I knew in my heart that the problem wasn't in my teeth. The pain would move and at times seemed to be in my gums or on the left side of my face. When I couldn't get any answers from the dentists, I began to research online other potential causes of unexplained mouth and facial pain, such as sinus infection, heart disease, brain tumor, multiple sclerosis, trigeminal neuralgia, and more. This just made me feel worse!

28

"My dentist decided that the next step was to see a neurologist. I ended up seeing two neurologists and having various tests. The only thing the tests showed was a little sinus congestion. After all the tests were completed, the neurologist concluded that my pain was most likely caused by an overactive nerve in my mouth and he prescribed two medications for nerve pain. He also referred me to an ear, nose, and throat specialist to look into the sinus congestion.

"The nerve medications didn't help, nor did the visit with the ENT. I felt as if I was losing a grip on my life. I have a 4-year-old daughter with special needs, and it upset me very much that I had to rely on my husband, mother, and nanny to take her to school and care for her. Two months had passed and I was still in pain and losing hope that I was going to get better. While I was getting more and more frustrated, I was still determined to get rid of the pain. I even tried lying in bed for a week, thinking that if I just rested and didn't use my mouth, maybe that would help. It didn't. The most painful thing, however, was watching my family live life without me. I mentioned my problem to a friend who suggested that I see a dentist who was a facial pain doctor."

Why were Jane's previous doctors and dentists unable to accurately diagnosis her problem? What made it so difficult? Without a full understanding of pain mechanisms in the facial region, dentists and physicians are limited in their ability to provide effective treatment. As a result, patients often become less confident that they can be helped. In extreme circumstances, practitioners send patients away, telling them such things as "Your pain is not real," "It's all in your head," "There's nothing wrong and you'll just have to live with it," or "It will go away." It is not uncommon for such patients to be referred to us with an apology from the referring doctors that "These patients are crazy."

## Key Pain-Related Factors that Account for Patient Misdiagnosis

Patients with facial-related pain and discomfort are misunderstood and misdiagnosed due to three key factors:

1.    Facial pain is commonly caused by a "distant" source, that is, the source of the pain is not near the location of the actual pain site. This phenomenon, called referred pain, was discussed at some length in Chapter 2.

2.    The intensity of facial pain often prompts patients and doctors to look for serious causes—which leads to extensive consultation and diagnostic testing in the search for disease, illness, or structural deficits—rather than to focus on the most common source of the pain, muscles. Without a full understanding of how muscle compromise can lead to persistent and debilitating facial pain problems, healthcare providers are often baffled by their patients' pain symptoms, and are unable to make an accurate diagnosis or provide effective treatment.

3.    Although researchers well understand the biological mechanisms by which emotions prompt the onset of muscle tension and facial pain, dental and medical practitioners involved in patient care are either uncomfortable or are only partially effective in communicating this reality to their patients.

## Limits of Traditional Medical and Dental Training

As a result of the above three factors, facial pain problems, which could be diagnosed and readily managed, linger and continue to burden patients. One of the main reasons doctors and dentists generally lack diagnostic and treatment efficacy when it comes to understanding facial pain symptoms is a result of their professional training.

Even though the focus on pain education has improved over the years, the vast majority of today's dental and medical schools provide limited education and training in the area of chronic pain in general, and facial pain specifically. An editorial appropriately titled "Why Mouthless Medical Schools?" for example, which appeared several decades ago in the *New England Journal of Medicine* (Sognnaes, 1977) still rings true today. Physicians receive little or no education regarding the oral, dental, or temporomandibular structures, and essentially look through the oral cavity when examining the tonsils and adenoids. To them, patients are, thus, essentially "mouthless," as the title of the article suggests.

As for dentists, it is interesting to note that, historically, the dental profession has given limited attention to educating its students beyond the teeth and oral structures. In fact, even in dental schools today there is wide disparity in the content of the pain curricula. Some schools have developed separate departments that teach about facial pain, while others randomly assign pain topics to a variety of restorative dental disciplines but never provide a comprehensive approach to this area or concern. As a result, many students ultimately rely on a mechanistic/structural orientation with regard to the origin and management of facial pain problems when, in fact, the majority of patients with facial pain do not have major structural compromises or bad bites.

Though many dentists have broadened their education in assessing facial pain problems, they continue to have a structuralist approach when diagnosing and treating pain complaints. Many dentists in their attempt to solve facial pain problems focus on the patient's "bite," since that has traditionally been the thinking when it comes to understanding, diagnosing, and treating facial pain. This treatment approach, however, is not based on science. In fact, despite the common use of these mechanistic approaches, extensive research has failed to find a convincing connection between structural factors and facial pain (de Leeuw, 2008; Seligman & Pullinger, 1991). As a profession that has its foundations in tooth anatomy, it is not surprising that dentists normally take a structuralist and mechanistic approach to solving facial pain problems. Bite adjustments and tooth alterations are commonly used to treat facial pain, in spite of the fact that these measures have unpredictable outcomes and can create irreversible structural changes.

Since some common facial pain symptoms are due to readily diagnosed conditions in the teeth, sinuses, and salivary glands, it continues to be a challenge to get physicians and dentists to accept the possibility that similar pain symptoms that linger, despite treatment efforts, have their origins in *muscles*. Even when a tooth continues to hurt after a cavity is filled or a root canal procedure is done, or when a sinus is unresponsive to a wash-out procedure and several courses of antibiotics, dentists and physicians routinely continue to look for structural reasons for the pain. We have always found it fascinating that a dental x-ray, which typically can be viewed and judged in 10-15 seconds, is often scrutinized for minutes when a patient has a lingering facial pain problem.

In all fairness, many physicians and dentists refuse to treat symptoms when no discernable physical findings are uncovered, but their reluctance to explain to patients how their physical symptoms may have an emotional or psychological origin remains a problem. Also, medical and dental practitioners commonly make judgments based on the level of pain a patient is experiencing. The intensity of pain, however, does not necessarily correlate with the seriousness of a problem. Pain that patients report as "intense" often leads to extensive testing and evaluation based on the conclusion that there is a serious problem. For most of our patients, however, this is not the case.

In addition to pain severity, dentists and physicians often view patients' symptoms that seemly have a nerve origin as indicating a serious medical problem. A complaint of "My face tingles and feels numb," for example, is often evaluated with serious rigor, though the symptoms may simply be a result of tight muscles that create a slight decrease in the level of oxygen in the muscle tissues.

Full neurologic evaluations are certainly welcome and necessary at times, but when testing does not give rise to a specific diagnosis, it is insufficient for a doctor to say, "Don't worry it will go away with time," without providing some discussion as to why there are symptoms in the absence of disease. Without insight into a patient's psychosocial history, the possibility that the pain could be a result of problems with the muscles is often left out of the discussion. Patients worry, therefore, despite repeated assurances that they are not sick.

## Lack of Conversation and Misdiagnosis

As the above discussion suggests, another reason facial pain problems are often misdiagnosed is because many physicians and dentists minimize the importance of taking a detailed personal and psychosocial history of the patient—especially one that includes the challenges and conflicts the patient faces on a daily basis. In most cases, the time healthcare professionals spend with patients has diminished significantly over the years, as a result of complex issues facing our medical system. Patient evaluations commonly focus only on the body part that is hurting—a narrow approach that often produces an inaccurate diagnosis.

## Philosophical Biases and Misdiagnosis

Patients often assume they are in pain because of a structural flaw in their body. Commonly they express sentiments such as "I have back pain because of my scoliosis," "My neck hurts because my spine curvature is too straight," or "My face hurts because I have a bad bite." Many people, including healthcare professionals, believe that the loss of body symmetry is the reason for the onset or persistence of pain symptoms. This is not the case, however. Although patients frequently have come to our offices convinced that their facial pain is due to structural factors such as neck curvature, uneven shoulder heights, altered bite relations, or an asymmetric position of the jaw, no credible scientifically-based study has identified these factors as a specific cause of facial muscle pain.

Unfortunately, despite this lack of credible support, medical and dental practitioners often misinform and misguide patients based on philosophical biases. These biases are established and supported by convincing arguments presented at continuing education seminars, in journal articles, or on the Internet. Once established, they are hard to shake, and physicians often embrace them when patients are looking for a solution to their pain. Although we do not discount the possibility that these structural deviations could contribute to facial pain, a survey of large dental populations suggests that they are not causal. If men and women both have these structural deviations, then why is it that approximately 80% of the patients we see are women? In addition, a survey of patients with "bad bites" commonly seen in dental practices clearly reveals that there are just as many who do not have any pain symptoms as there are who are in pain. How could this be if structural issues were truly the cause of facial pain?

## Consequences of Misdiagnosis

As a result of misdiagnosis and ineffective treatment of facial pain problems, patients' symptoms continue with profound consequences that negatively impact their lives in general. Patients might begin to limit their physical activities, for example, and avoid situations they believe will result in additional pain and suffering. Many people begin to cut their food into small pieces, or wait until mid-afternoon before eating, so their muscles have time to "warm up." Still others don't smile or yawn for fear of more pain. At times, patients have confided in us that they no longer enjoy kissing or sexual relations, as these activities increase their pain. They also avoid certain sleeping positions that bring the face in contact with the pillow, which affects their sleep.

As a result of these "pain behaviors," muscles can become even further compromised due to compensations, atrophy, or both, as normal function is avoided. Oddly enough, what often starts out as symptoms without a serious physical problem can progress to a more complex physical problem, as patients modify their behavior to avoid pain. As a result, the facial pain sufferer can end up with symptoms that have considerable variability.

## Summary

Patients are socialized to think of facial pain as resulting from injury, disease, a neurological problem, or a structural malfunction, and thus they seek out traditional practitioners for the perceived problem, e.g., a dentist for tooth pain or an ENT for an ear ache. Dentists, ENT specialists, neurologists, and other healthcare professionals are insufficiently prepared to properly diagnose most types or causes of facial pain, however, because of the nature of their training. Medical schools, for example, largely ignore the mouth and jaw, and most healthcare professionals have not been trained to even consider emotions as part of their diagnoses, let alone discuss that dimension of human life with their patients. As a result of these gaps in their professional training, what most healthcare professionals typically look for when patients report either facial pain or other symptoms—such as odd sensations or functional problems in their facial region—are signs of structural problems, injury, trauma to tissues, nerve disorders, or disease. Because the great majority of healthcare professionals do not understand the true cause of most facial pain (once toothaches have been eliminated), their treatments often fail to bring relief to patients. As a result, patients waste much money and time, suffer unnecessary frustration, and are puzzled as to what to do next. This confusion often results in patients losing hope and developing sleep problems, heightened anxiety, and various negative emotions that further exacerbate their facial-related problems.

## Chapter 5

# THE TRUE CAUSE OF MOST PERSISTENT FACIAL PAIN: MUSCLES AND THE "BRAIN UNDER SIEGE"

*The face is the mirror of the mind, and eyes without speaking confess the secrets of the heart.* — St. Jerome

In the body as a whole, muscles are essentially responsible for every movement you make, from the moment you open your eyes in the morning until you put your head on the pillow at night. This is so whether your movements are voluntary, such as turning your head or chewing, or involuntary (i.e., automatic), such as breathing or the beating of your heart. First, movements are initiated as your brain sends messages to specific muscle groups. Once a muscle has been called upon to perform a specific action, the brain then monitors and regulates the completion of that action. We take the smooth and efficient functioning of muscles for granted, but normal, pain-free muscle activity occurs only if there is consistent regulation of the neural and circulatory systems that support muscle health.

The human face, as previously mentioned, is mainly comprised of muscles. Therefore, if you have facial pain that is persistent, the reason for the pain is probably a fatigued and over-contracted muscle in your facial area or neck. In addition, problems may also occur in one or more of the structures associated with the muscles, such as nerves, ligaments, and tendons.

But why do your muscles hurt? What is the source that produces the pain in your muscles? We believe the answer, in most cases—but not all—is actually your emotions, i.e., your psycho-emotional state, which is created and influenced by life events and circumstances. That conclusion may be difficult for you to contemplate upon first hearing it, unless you understand and accept the concept of a "mind-body connection." This connection is often referred to as a psychophysiologic (Laskin,1982) or *pychosomatic* explanation of physical pain (Sarno, 2006). Without such an understanding and acceptance, you may naturally ask yourself, "How can emotions be the source of pain in my muscles, and if they are, is it possible for me to feel better though my world may be difficult to change?"

For you to fully understand how the mind-body connection works as it relates to facial pain, you first need to have a clear picture of the muscles in the face and neck and how they function in a pain-free manner, which is the goal of the first part this chapter. Once you have this picture and knowledge firmly in mind, you will be able to understand how your psycho-emotional state can often cause a *physical change* in your muscles—both directly and through learned behaviors—as well as in the nerves that run through all muscle tissue. Conveying this information is the goal of the second part of this chapter. You may be surprised to learn that if you understand and accept the explanation presented in this chapter, and begin to change learned behaviors that have developed as a result of emotions, your facial pain may suddenly lessen or even disappear!

## The Muscular Makeup of Your Face, Head and Neck: All You Need To Know

The muscles of the face, head, and neck are shown in the figures on the following two pages. Figure 4 shows the muscles of facial expression, Figure 5 shows the muscles of mastication (used for chewing), and Figure 6 shows the cervical (or neck) muscles. These muscles are skeletal muscles that are under the conscious control of the brain. When they and their associated structures (nerves, tendons, and ligaments) are working properly and are perfectly in "sync," they perform a multitude of tasks, both independently and in concert.

The muscles of the face and neck are responsible for your ability to open and close your eyes and mouth, smile, kiss, chew, and perform a multitude of other movements, such as drink, swallow, speak, and turn your head in different directions.

Figure 4: Muscles of Facial Expression

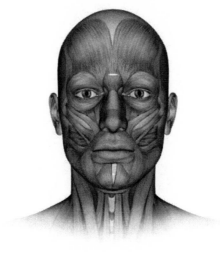

Figure 5: Muscles of Mastication

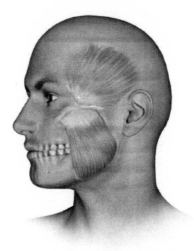

Figure 6: Cervical Muscles

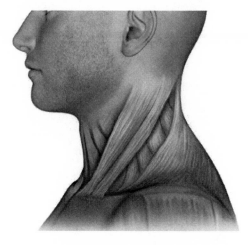

## The "Automatic" Actions of Facial Muscles and the Brain

We take these everyday facial actions for granted and don't give this region a second thought when all is working well. Think about the simple activity of eating, for example. Without conscious thought or awareness, the first stage of digestion requires careful choreography of the tongue, cheek, and jaw muscles, and the input of sensory nerve endings in the lining of the mouth and the ligament attachments of teeth to bone. We chew an apple, bite a carrot, or reduce steak into a digestible mass by moving the food from side to side without conscious direction from the brain, until the food is smooth enough to be swallowed. The mouth knows how to operate based on the wetness, dryness, hardness, and consistency of the food. The oral apparatus can automatically detect small fish bones amidst a mouthful of food, and the jaw knows the amount of pressure to exert to break food into small pieces in a reflex manner without thought or planning. These precise activities are programmed into the brain as a result of repetition and the healthy functioning of muscles, nerves, temporomandibular (TM) joints, and other structures of the mouth.

## *The Tale of the Two Saltine Crackers*

A demonstration we did with high school students illustrates in a very simple way how the automatic "detection devices" of the mouth and jaw work. Two groups of students were given two dry saltine crackers and told to take only two bites and then to swallow. Both groups tried to swallow the crackers when asked to, but could not. Then both groups were given two more crackers and this time they were instructed to continue to chew until they were told to swallow. After 15 or 20 bites, the students could no longer suppress the need to swallow.

When the students asked us what was going on, we explained that there were "detection devices" attached to the teeth and in the lining of the mouth and tongue that were providing the brain with the information needed to know when it was safe to swallow the crackers to protect the mouth and esophagus. All that the brain needed to know was the wetness of the crackers and the particle size to signal "continue to chew" or "stop chewing and swallow."

From this simple experiment, you can see how your muscles and facial structures, when they are functioning normally, coordinate with your brain automatically to accomplish critical activities that we take for granted every day, like the simple act of eating a cracker.

## Energy and Muscle Pain

All muscles require energy to perform efficiently. The energy in muscles, called ATP (for Adenosine-5'-triphosphate), is continually being replenished during the course of one's life. If the muscles have an insufficient amount of ATP stored in them, then they often feel weak, tired, and sore, and normal functions are compromised.

A critical point to remember in this context is that it takes the same amount of energy, or ATP molecules, to contract a muscle as it does to relax it. If it takes 10 units of energy, for example, to make a fist with your hand, then it will take 10 units of energy for you to disengage the fist and return your hand to a relaxed, resting position. If all the available energy is utilized to make and maintain the fist, then there will not be a sufficient amount of energy left to relax the fist fully, and a sensation of tension and fatigue—and perhaps pain—will be felt in the hand.

The same phenomenon applies to the jaw. If, for example, the normal amount of energy available to the jaw muscles is depleted due to continuous contracture, the jaw will not be able to return to its normal resting position or assume normal functions. In essence, when the energy resources in jaw muscles are depleted, normal muscle function is impossible, and even resting postures, like keeping the teeth apart, will require conscious thought and effort.

Quite often we see patients who tell us that even when they are on vacation their pain does not lessen. The reason is undoubtedly that, even though their physical environment changes, these patients take their unique muscle-bracing tendencies with them, and therefore create continued contracture and deplete critical reserves of energy. Unless patients stop over-utilizing their muscles, they are destined for continued suffering.

## Muscles and Their Related Structures

### Fascia and Muscles

Muscles are composed of individual fibers that are each wrapped in a thin, tight sheath of connective tissue known as fascia (see Figure 7 on page 41). Fascia creates a wrapping around muscles, much like a sausage casing, and it provides muscles with structural support and protection. It is like a big cobweb that interconnects muscle tissue and is molded according to the pattern of muscle use.

If a muscle is either overworked or continually in a state of contracture, the fascia surrounding and permeating the muscle becomes tight and restricted. This can prevent the muscle from accomplishing the work it is designed to do, by inhibiting the full release and relaxation of the tight muscle. In addition, when fascial tissue becomes twisted or bound around a nerve in a band of muscle, the nerve can become irritated until symptoms such as pain, tingling, burning, and weakness are experienced. These fascial alterations can occur as a result of repetitive activities that strain the muscles, physical trauma, and chronic emotional turmoil.

If muscles are contracted for an extended period of time, then their energy reserves become depleted, as explained above. Once energy stores are depleted, restoration to a normal level will only occur if there is an adequate supply of oxygen and nutrients. This will not happen if the muscle tissues remain contracted and the associated fascia is altered.

Figure 7: Fascial Web that Interconnects Muscle Tissue

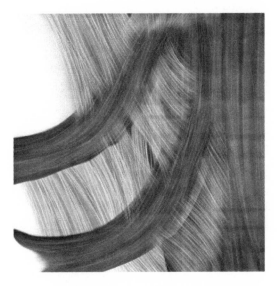

## Tendons and Muscles

Tendons connect muscles to the surrounding boney architecture of the head, face, neck, and other bodily areas. When muscles begin to falter, it is likely that with time their associated tendons will become compromised and contribute to the emergence and perpetuation of symptoms. When tendons are functioning normally, they receive less blood flow, oxygen, and nutrients than muscle fibers, and so they have less capacity to repair themselves. Once they are compromised, therefore, healing is even more difficult. It is common for our facial pain patients to place their fingers directly over boney areas where the tendons of several muscles attach, when they are asked to identify where they hurt most. Since some of these tendon sites can only be felt in the mouth, patients routinely stick their fingers in their mouth to make sure we understand where they hurt.

**Tendonitis.** Where tendons exist in the face, such as in the jaw, tendonitis can occur. Just like tendonitis responsible for so-called "tennis elbow" (purportedly from overuse of the elbow), tendonitis in the jaw muscles can occur due to overutilization. Persistent tooth contact, clenching, nail and cuticle biting, and even aggressive gum chewing, which we see in patients who attempt to cope with intense job stress, can bring on tendonitis and pain. It is, therefore, critical to remember that since the jaw is an orthopedic apparatus, its use must be respected if comfort and normal function is to be preserved.

## Nerves, Ligaments, and Muscles

Running through all muscles are nerve fibers. They are the "messengers" that carry information (or "signals") from the muscles to the brain and from the brain to the muscles. The information transmitted through nerves regulate the tension and length of the muscles. As nerve fibers are directly influenced by the chemical environment of muscle tissue, it is not uncommon for these nerves to fire excessively as a result of muscle compromise. This excessive nerve activity travels back to the brain and the experience of pain is triggered.

Just as muscles can affect nerve activity, excessive nerve excitation that begins in the brain can influence muscles in the face and neck. If messages (electrical activity) coming from the brain via nerves have been heightened, for example, the messages may cause muscles to contract or change their tone, thus altering performance capacity and comfort.

Nerve fibers are not only found in muscles, but also in the periodontal ligaments that connect the teeth to the supporting bone of the jaws. The nerve receptors (proprioceptors) in these ligaments are responsible for the signals that are sent to the brain during activities like chewing or nonfunctional tooth contact. When you bring your teeth together after a dentist has put in a restoration, it is the proprioceptors in the periodontal ligaments that inform the brain whether or not that restoration is too high and requires additional adjustment.

In like fashion, when you are eating a meal, the nerves in the periodontal ligaments detect the texture and density of the food, and are responsible for making the muscles ease off or work harder to chew the food into a form that is capable of being swallowed. The nerve endings in these ligaments are designed for quick judgments, not sustained functioning, such as that required to provide continuous signals back to the brain. In a patient who frequently brings her teeth together or who often checks her bite (to see if the teeth are fitting properly), these nerve endings take on a new role, which they are not accustomed to handling efficiently.

Patients with a tendency to overutilize the jaw and bring the teeth together frequently excite the nerve endings of the periodontal ligaments excessively, and thereby contribute to the onset of facial pain problems. Figure 8 below shows the tooth pulp and the periodontal ligament that surrounds it. The pulp is the dark mass in the center of the tooth and the periodontal ligament is the curved structure around the outside bottom area of the pulp, which ends at the apex (indicated by the horizontal line at the bottom of the figure).

Figure 8: Periodontal Ligament

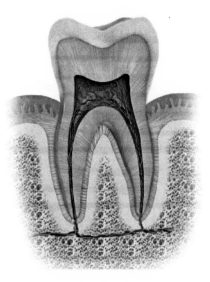

## "Sprinters" and "Long Distance Runners": Two Types of Muscles

The role of muscles can vary in terms of "tension," ranging from long-term maintenance of tension, e.g., to support your head, to brief periods of tension, e.g., when you are eating or expressing an emotion with a smile or a grimace. Some muscles, in other words, are designed for short-term activity and other muscles are designed for sustained function. Muscles designed for short-term activity are called fast-twitch muscles, or "sprinters," such as the jaw muscles. Muscles designed for sustained function are called slow-twitch muscles, or "long distance runners," such as the neck muscles. Each of these muscle groups is designed to perform specific tasks. When they are asked to participate in activities for which they were not designed, then muscle function and efficiency are significantly reduced, and pain is likely to result.

## Facial Expressions and Muscles

The muscles of facial expression (see Figure 4, p. 37) are "sprinters," and are most recognizable because they are responsible for smiling, frowning, lip puckering, and the numerous other emotions you express on a daily basis. Like all muscles, they are designed to function in specific ways, resting with normal tone and contracting when called to action. Your state of mind has a great deal of influence over which of these muscles are active and how long they are active.

When we experience emotional turmoil and distress, it is often evident in our facial expressions and the ways in which we hold tension in our facial muscles. As you now know, when this tension is ongoing and your brain becomes overwhelmed, it can lead to muscle fatigue, soreness, and, eventually, pain. If you remember a happy experience when you smiled all day for the camera, for example, the day you were married or graduated from college, you can appreciate how sore and painful the facial muscles can be after sustained use. In a similar fashion, the emotions of sadness, loneliness, desperation and anger can engage these muscles in persistent postures of tension that lead to pain.

Mara was a patient who illustrates the symptoms that can result when the muscles of facial expression get fatigued from remaining in the same position or posture over an extended period of time. As soon as Mara sat down in the consultation room, it was obvious she had a "forced smile" continually on her face. She carried a large briefcase, was dressed in a suit, and her perpetual smile spread from ear to ear. It turned out, as suspected, that she was a "drug rep," a pharmaceutical salesperson. Her tight smile didn't leave her face for one minute. Before she had the opportunity to describe what troubled her, it was apparent why her face ached all day. Mara's appearance and demeanor made the diagnosis easy, and she did not dispute it. Her desire to appear friendly and accessible, the "super salesperson," required her to maintain a smile on her face at all times, regardless of how she was feeling, which was actually tense and nervous about making her sales quota. When this was pointed out to her, she immediately relaxed her face and expressed relief at the simple prescription offered: Avoid tensing those muscles for long periods of time and your pain will go away.

## The Jaw Muscles

The muscles of mastication (see figure 5, page 37) dominate the face, and are either fully or partly responsible for opening and closing the mouth, chewing, swallowing, speaking, and breathing. They are "sprinters," and essentially responsible for all jaw function. To fully understand how these muscles can dominate individuals' experience of pain problems in the face and jaw, it is important to understand how the jaw works.

The lower jaw is a V-shaped bone suspended in space. It is attached to the bones of the skull at each end by the temporomandibular (TM) joints, and maintains a certain posture and position against the pull of gravity. This position is established by the tension of several pairs of muscles. When the jaw is at rest and hanging slack, the upper and lower teeth are apart, with the air freely flowing between the teeth. This "freeway space" is usually maintained during one's waking hours. For some people the upper and lower teeth do come together during swallowing, but that is usually only for a brief instant before they go back to their resting posture. These periods of brief tooth contact do not overutilize, fatigue, or injure jaw muscles.

When the jaw is in this open, relaxed position, blood flow is sustained, bringing fresh oxygen and nutrients to the muscles, the attachment tendons, and the nerve fibers that run throughout the muscles. An adequate supply of oxygen and nutrition is required by the muscles in order to remain healthy and to function, based on the design created during embryologic development.

The major muscles in the jaw region, as mentioned above, are the fast-twitch sprinters. They are designed for short-term activities like chewing and speaking, which involve quick and spontaneous actions and, therefore, do not require an ongoing supply of energy. The chewing muscles (muscles of mastication) typically are not engaged in action for more than several minutes three to four times a day. When healthy, these muscles bring the teeth together consistently so that food can be chewed in an efficient and predictable way. During speaking, normal muscle tone allows the jaw and the tongue to move in complex and subtle ways for smooth and unimpeded conversation.

You can think of the jaw as a bus and the teeth and tongue as passengers. If the position of the jaw is altered even slightly due to fatigued jaw muscles or muscles that are holding excess tension, then the teeth will not come together in a normal fashion, prompting patients to experience symptoms such as "My teeth don't fit like they used to," "My teeth clash when I chew," or "My bite is off balance." If the position of the tongue has been influenced by an altered jaw position, then patients often say their speech has changed or they can't pronounce certain sounds as they did in the past.

Within the mouth, the teeth function only to help shape the sounds of speech and, of course, to participate in the grinding, ripping, and tearing of food during the chewing process. The muscles provide the source of power and the teeth are the cutting surfaces. As long as muscles are healthy and there are enough teeth to do the gripping, milling, and grinding of food, then the chewing process occurs in a reflex fashion. Most of us never give any thought to how food is broken down in the mouth and swallowed. In fact, it is normal for us to eat and carry on conversation at the same time. It is only when our muscles and the TM joints do not function properly that we become aware of the chewing process.

If there are muscles that close the jaws, to bring the teeth together, then there also must be muscles that open the jaws, to allow common actions like yawning to occur. In addition, there are jaw muscles that allow movements from side to side and forward and back, as the teeth are kept apart.

All of these muscles are part of the group called the muscles of mastication, and they play a unique role in normal jaw function. When functioning properly, these muscles help support normal activity of the jaw without pain. When these muscles are fatigued, however, or over-contracted and tense, they can impact jaw movements and often place strain on the TM joints.

When sprinter jaw muscles are shortened to bring the teeth together for long periods of time, as in clenching or persistent daytime tooth contact, they cannot function properly. Over time they become tired and sore, and are the focus of many of our facial pain patients.

This is what happened with Robin, a 29-year-old mother with two young children, who was clearly in trouble when she arrived at the office. Robin came accompanied by her mother, for support and to make sure she remembered the details of her story. Within a few minutes, it was clear that she was, as she put it, "at the end of her rope." Robin had been suffering from ear pain for the past 8 months, and on this particular day her pain was particularly severe. She suspected that the rainy weather was responsible. As reported by many of our patients, Robin said her pain came on spontaneously without a specific triggering event or provoking factor. Her pain had prompted eight professional consultations, and although she had been assured that she did not have a terrible medical problem, she had not been given a specific diagnosis or hope that her symptoms would go away.

As the mother of two young children, 1 and 3 years old, Robin "had no time for the pain." Because her pain made her very tired and changed her cheery disposition by the end of the day, she felt that she was struggling to meet her family's needs. Her mother described her as a high-strung, highly stressed, tense person who did not know how to relax, but Robin countered by saying that she had a great life, great kids, and a great husband. Just at that moment, Robin's facial muscles bulged. From talking with her, it became clear that her teeth were constantly in contact or she was biting her tongue, lip, or cuticles as she went about her daily routine. In essence, Robin's daytime tendencies had taken sprinters and required them to become long-distance runners. As a result, her jaw muscles were fatigued and likely contributing to her ear pain due to the mechanisms responsible for referred pain (see Chapter 2 for a discussion of referred pain).

## TM Joints and Muscles

The temporomandibular joints (TMJs) play an important role in all jaw movements. These two "jaw joints" are located right in front of your ears and connect the ends of the V-shaped lower jaw to the bones of the skull (see Figure 9, page 48). They are the hinges that make it possible for the lower jaw to be opened and closed and moved from side to side and forward and back, performing a multitude of functions on a daily basis. It is the connection of the right and left joints on one bone that makes this joint system different from those in the elbows or knees. Whatever happens to one temporomandibular joint must influence the other.

The TM joints are lubricated with synovial fluid, as are most joints in the body. This fluid also provides nourishment for the joints, and an adequate supply of synovial fluid is essential for the health of these joints. Synovial fluid volume is kept at normal levels when jaw motion is relatively normal and the jaw has full capacity to move in all directions without hindrance or compromise.

Figure 9: The Temporomandibular Joint

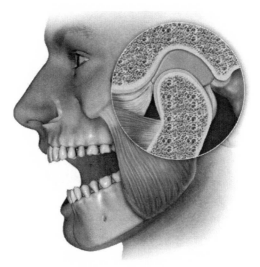

In a healthy jaw joint system, droplets of synovial fluid are deposited in the joints on a consistent basis, due to what is known as weeping lubrication. The synovial fluid maintains contact with the joint structures due to a sac-like structure called a capsule. Within this capsule, we find the lower part of the joint, called the mandibular condyle, and a disc or piece of cartilage, which is a "shock absorber" held in place by ligaments that bind this cartilage to the condyle and other boney structures in this area.

When the mouth is opened and closed, and the jaws move, the cartilage moves with the condyle, much like your hand on a stick shift. As long as the ligaments are intact and the shape of the cartilage remains in its normal form, an intimate contact remains between all the elements. If, however, the ligaments are stretched, the cartilage shape changes, or both, there is the potential for slipping of the cartilage, leading to symptoms such as locking and clicking, popping, and gravelly types of sounds. The synovial fluid plays a critical role in maintaining the shape of the cartilage and nourishing the ligaments so that they maintain their integrity.

## TM Joints and Muscles Work Together

The muscles and the TM joints work together and, as with all muscle-joint collaborations, there is the potential for breakdown of the joints. Problems with the TM joints lead to complaints and symptoms of pain, limited motion, and joint noise.

Since the muscles of the jaw are responsible for moving the TM joints, when problems occur in the muscles, joint movement will be affected. The reverse is also true. If there are independent problems in the joint, the muscles will react in one way or another and their performance will be compromised. As we saw with the relationship between nerves and muscles, problems can move in both directions.

## TM Dysfunction

The term "temporomandibular dysfunction," or TMD, has been defined as "a collection of medical and dental conditions affecting the TMJ and/or the muscles of mastication, as well as associated structures" (NIH consensus statement, 1986). From our perspective. these conditions are essentially orthopedic problems and, as a result, are often associated with signs and symptoms common to compromised joints and muscles throughout the body. Though a TMD problem may only involve muscles, it has been our preference through the years to assign a TMD diagnosis only when there is evidence of mechanical problems in the TM joints that lead to symptoms of joint pain, persistent bite changes, and/or complaints of joint clicking, popping or locking. It should, therefore, be understood that the population of patients described in this book, who have facial pain of muscle origin, may be identified as having a TMD problem by other clinicians.

## Facial Pain and Neck Muscles

To fully understand facial pain problems, it is necessary to know about the muscles of the neck (see Figure 6, page 38). They determine and maintain head posture and are responsible for the rotation, extension, and side movements of the head. Attached to the spine, these muscles resist the downward pull of gravity while maintaining the upright posture required for the head during our waking hours. In this role, they have a profound impact on the posture and position of the lower jaw.

While the jaw muscles are sprinters, neck muscles are long distance runners, as they are called into action for extended periods of time during one's waking hours. Based on our encounters with facial pain patients over the years, it is our opinion that a large proportion of them have facial symptoms that originate in the muscles of the neck.

When the neck muscles are fatigued or abnormally tense, as a result of ongoing emotional challenges and anguish, they can give rise to a number of symptoms, including generalized facial pain, jaw tension, ear pain, eye pressure, clogged ears, bite discrepancies, temporal and frontal headaches, diminished jaw motion, and facial tingling and numbness. These symptoms may develop spontaneously or accompany changes in head position while one is lying down, sitting at work, or simply attending to everyday activities. For the most part, the jaw and other facial symptoms that arise from the neck come on slowly, in the absence of an identifiable event. Many of our patients, however, are in the midst of emotional turmoil or have come through significant life events, which we believe most likely triggered over-contraction and fatigue of the neck muscles.

Rick was a patient whose life circumstances led to facial pain that originated in the muscles of the neck. He presented with intense right facial pain that would begin in the morning and linger all day. His neck was tense and periodically he developed tingling in his fingers. In addition, he felt that his back teeth were not fitting, but if he chewed gum for several minutes, his teeth would meet in a more consistent way and his facial pain would ease a bit. Within several minutes after chewing, however, his symptoms would slowly re-emerge.

Rick said he had these symptoms for approximately 4 weeks. With questioning, he revealed that he had been going through a divorce and had two young children, 6 and 8 years old. About 10 days prior to coming for diagnosis, his wife had him arrested. She told the police that Rick had assaulted her when he refused to leave the apartment while visiting their children. Recalling this event, Rick remembered that he experienced numbness in his fingers and tension in his neck as he was being taken to the station house.

An examination revealed normal jaw motion and only minor discomfort when the right side of his face and jaw was palpated (examined by touch with gentle pressure to determine the level of tightness and tenderness). When the right side of his neck and shoulder was palpated, however, Rick experienced exquisite pain, and his right facial pain symptoms increased markedly. Clearly, it appeared that Rick's symptoms had their origin in the muscles of the upper neck and shoulder region. According to our mind-body explanatory model (which is discussed shortly below in detail), Rick's anger and anxiety gave rise to altered physiology in these muscles and, in turn, to the ultimate emergence of symptoms, as the jaw muscles were forced into a state of contracture. With supportive muscle treatment and understanding—about how an upset brain was more than capable of changing muscle physiology—Rick improved considerably.

Rick never really had a jaw problem. His facial symptoms occurred as a result of dysfunctional neck muscles that prompted his jaw and other facial muscles to be held in a tense posture. His need to chew gum to ease his pain (which actually pumped fresh blood and oxygen into his tense jaw muscles) was no longer necessary. Rick was discharged from treatment and his yearly holiday cards, with his two smiling children on the cover, clearly indicated that he understood and took to heart the suggestions we offered.

## Mechanisms Involved in Neck Muscles and Facial Pain

Complex neurological processes are responsible for the mechanisms that directly allow neck muscles to produce facial pain. The first process, called muscle co-contracture, is responsible for irritated, fatigued and painful neck muscles initiating the shortening of the jaw muscles responsible for all jaw movements. Though no specific insult has been sustained by the jaw muscles, the shortening of these muscle fibers leads to pain and an often bewildered patient. The second process involves the mechanism of referred pain, which we previously introduced. Research has demonstrated that muscles that allow movement (skeletal muscles)—including those in the neck—have the capacity to refer pain or other symptoms. This phenomenon is similar to the referral of pain to the left arm during a heart attack. The referred pain that results from skeletal muscles is often dull and aching, but it can increase and become acute when the responsible muscles are stimulated by repeated muscle contractions. Other symptoms that may appear due to referral mechanisms are often vague in their character and can change from moment to moment.

The diagnostic confusion that arises from referral mechanisms that are not understood leads to even greater patient anxiety and worry. Bigger problems arise, however, when treatment is directed at the location of the pain, as opposed to its true origin. Unfortunately, this was the case for 56-year-old Grace, a patient who had been in pain for almost 2 years.

Grace came to the office with symptoms of ongoing jaw, ear, and other facial pain. Her pain was dominant on the right side and varied daily in intensity and responsiveness to over-the-counter medication. She had been evaluated and treated by her primary care physician and two otolaryngologists, but her symptoms remained unresponsive to antibiotics and a host of other medications to clear congestion and alleged sinus inflammation. Dental and oral surgery consultations suggested a TMJ disorder. Neither the use of a bite appliance nor adjustment of her bite teeth produced a benefit, however. A consultation with a neurologist prompted a diagnosis of a facial migraine. When the prescribed medication made her sick to her stomach, she stopped taking it.

Although Grace had no neck complaints, examination of her neck muscles prompted a cry of pain and this comment: "I never knew those muscles were so sore." A more comprehensive evaluation revealed that the upper neck muscles were indeed excessively tight. Continued examination of these areas increased her jaw and other facial pain. It was clear that Grace's complaints of pain had their origins in the neck muscles.

As we would expect, in keeping with our explanatory model, additional questioning revealed a personal landscape strewn with life experiences and circumstances that likely compromised her brain's ability to maintain normal neural, circulatory, and muscle functioning. Not only had she lost her husband in the 9/11 tragedy, but her eldest daughter had been hospitalized for severe anxiety and depression. In addition, she was a colon cancer survivor and woke up every day worrying that the cancer would return.

Despite the depths of her suffering, it took just 3 months of treatment to reduce her pain and suffering to a marked degree. Grace's world had not changed, but her understanding of the referral mechanisms that initiated the pain, coupled with treatment directed at the implicated muscles, was all it took to initiate the recovery process.

*

As you have seen in the above discussion, the muscles and related structures of the face, head, and neck work together in exquisite collaboration to perform a multitude of tasks that include chewing, swallowing, smiling, speaking, opening and closing your mouth, and turning your head in different directions. Though seemingly simple, these tasks are actually quite complex, but they occur smoothly and effortlessly in a healthy muscle system. As we shall now explain, a brain "under siege" is all it takes for harmony to be disrupted and symptoms to emerge.

## Muscles and the Brain Under Siege: The Psycho-Emotional Basis of Facial Pain

The facial and neck muscles, which are responsible for both movement and maintaining certain positions or postures, can contract (i.e., shorten and tighten) quickly and powerfully, but when tired require rest in order to continue to function in a predictable, pain-free way. In most of our patients, the facial muscles ache continuously during the day, with higher levels of pain experienced when the muscles are called to action (e.g., for smiling, yawning, or eating).

The symptoms of facial pain most often develop, in other words, because the muscles of the neck and face are either on the verge of spasm or are gradually becoming more and more tense, fatigued, and sore. In this state, they are incapable of maintaining normal pain-free function. Now let us begin to explore the reasons why.

## Stress and the Brain Under Siege

Among the many and diverse patients we have seen over the years, we rarely have identified the source of their facial pain as coming from a single injury, a disease, or a structural or neurological problem. For this reason, we have concluded that the most likely cause of these common pain problems is the brain's inability to maintain normal neural and muscle function when under the persistent influence of factors such as anxiety and worry, constant conflicts and tensions, and difficult life circumstances. In addition, many of the people we see put a great deal of pressure on themselves, constantly demanding excellence and achievement in all they do. When the stress level becomes too high for individuals and they experience significant emotional reactions, especially for an extended period of time, we describe them as having a brain "under siege."

To better understand this concept, Dr. Kurt Olsson, a facial pain researcher, coined the term "The Emotional Motor Center" in 1996 to help explain how input to the brain directs daily human physiology and drives muscle activity. Dr. Olsson was essentially referring to the concept that what we see, hear, and smell creates thoughts and emotions that not only dictate muscle tension, but also generate muscle behaviors.

## Society-Wide Sources of Stress

Today, tens of millions of Americans—and hundreds of millions of people around the world—are experiencing stress from societal factors such as divorce, the death of a loved one, unemployment, severe sickness, caring for elderly parents, and financial insecurity, among many others. These societal conditions—which we may term "macro-sociological" factors—are sources of significant stress for teenagers and seniors as well as for an unprecedented number of adults, who are in the prime of their income-earning lives and responsible for taking care of their elderly parents and children simultaneously.

In this context, it should be reiterated that although most of our patients have been women (see Chapter 3), a brain under siege and overwhelming stress of any kind can be the catalyst for pain in men as well as in women. It is our impression that men tend to experience pain and other problems most often when they have financial problems, feel that they're losing control over the future and, especially, when they feel they cannot fulfill their most important role, taking care of their family. Men do not have the understanding necessary, any more than women do, to recognize why they are in pain and, as a result, anxiety sets in to make the problem worse. David was a patient whose case illustrates this well.

Fifty-three-year-old David had symptoms that included facial tension, tightness and pulling in the temporalis region, soreness in the hairline region, and a constant sense of discomfort in the jaw and face on the right side. He had these symptoms every day, though some days and weeks were better than others for no apparent reason. Overall however, he was becoming frustrated by his varied symptoms. David also had multiple sclerosis. When asked how he was coping with the knowledge that he had this disease, he described the impact of MS on his life. Essentially, he said, "From the moment I wake up I am aware that something is not quite right with me, and I'm worried about what the future will bring." He went on to explain that loss of control over his life made him constantly worry that he would not be able to meet his family's needs. Those worries, and that loss of control, it was clear, were at the root of David's facial pain.

## Personal Traumatic Events and Stress

In addition to macro-societal sources of stress, as discussed above, a careful review of the scientific literature reveals a startling statistic. In a number of controlled clinical studies, it has been shown that 50% to 64% of facial pain patients have experienced a profound traumatic event that preceded the onset of their pain. Specific traumatic events such as the death of a spouse, job loss, academic setbacks, military combat, or being the victim of rape, terrorism, or a natural disaster, as well as ongoing issues such as marital discord, illness, and physical or verbal abuse, have all been identified as significant precipitating factors of chronic pain.

## The Mind, Emotions, and Facial Pain

Based on our professional experience, evidence from research studies, case histories of patients, and the work of doctors such as John Sarno (1984, 1991, 2006), the author of several bestselling books on back pain, we believe that in most patients with facial pain the major cause of the pain is the mind and emotions—which can alter the chemical, physical, and biological state of muscles to the point where they hurt and don't function properly.

Long before contemporary researchers identified how the brain under siege could influence critical bodily functions, clinicians involved in taking care of patients with chronic pain believed that the emergence of physical symptoms had a psychological, or brain-related, origin. The term "psychophysiologic" process was coined to describe this relationship between the "psyche" and the body (Laskin & Greene, 1972). The theory suggests that factors that influence parts of the brain responsible for emotions are also ultimately responsible for initiating mechanisms that change the physiology and performance of organ systems.

This link can be seen in the case of Fran, who experienced a variety of symptoms in multiple body regions and organ systems as a result of psychophysiologic processes at work. When Fran first came for treatment some 15 years ago, she was 35 years old, married, and working as a nurse. She complained primarily of tightness in her face and jaw, and assumed this was due to her bad bite and a tendency to clench her teeth during the day. Questioning revealed that Fran was generally healthy, but often experienced gastrointestinal distress and, at times, anxiety attacks.

An examination did not reveal any profound compromise in her jaw structures, but there were multiple sites of pain across her jaw muscles, other facial muscles, and neck muscles. Also, her jaw muscles were well-developed and defined, which suggested longstanding nighttime clenching (bruxism) and frequent daytime tooth contact. As Fran suggested, she did, in fact, have a bite that could be classified as a malocclusion. Her lower jaw was positioned in front of her upper jaw and, as a result, her teeth did not hit evenly. Fran, however, had no problem chewing food and, in fact, at times found that chewing gum or food that had a heavy consistency would ease her facial pain symptoms.

Based on the supposition that Fran's symptoms had a muscular origin, she was put on a regimen of care that included techniques to relax her jaw during the day, an oral appliance at night, and facial exercises (see Chapter 6 for more on various treatment techniques). She was not treated for her malocclusion, however, since her teeth, though not aligned perfectly, were more than capable of normal chewing. Within a short period of time, Fran's symptoms diminished and she required only sporadic treatment, to make sure that her oral appliance was still in good condition.

Several years later, however, Fran returned for diagnosis and treatment after experiencing a major escalation of her symptoms. Not only did she have severe pain and tightness in her jaw and other facial muscles, she was most distressed by a new symptom of feeling off-balance. After multiple ear, nose, throat and neurology consultations, she was assured that there was no underlying disease, and was encouraged to return to her "TMJ doctor," because the other specialists believed her symptoms were likely due to her "bad bite."

Fran was convinced that, after all these years, her bad bite was truly at the heart of her suffering, and she showed her worn mouth guard as evidence. She was convinced that her pain would go away if her bite were fixed. Fran's evaluation, however, suggested otherwise, and pointed to the likelihood that sensitization mechanisms were playing a major role in her symptom experience. In fact, there was no other plausible explanation for the variety of symptoms she had in multiple body regions and organ systems, including gastrointestinal pain and frequent skin sensitivity. Her facial symptoms could not be explained by a malocclusion, and it was already clear that she did not have an underlying illness or disease. Why had things escalated so profoundly for Fran? Conversations with her provided the answers.

Over the years Fran's husband had taken ill, she had been transferred to work in a hospital located in an undesirable neighborhood, and, being a single child, she continued to worry about the health of her aging parents. Her brain was truly under siege and, as a result, a host of bodily symptoms developed and/or re-emerged at a more severe level. Fran had become one of those patients whose symptoms would be more difficult to manage because of her ongoing difficult life circumstances.

Although gender, sleep, and, in rare cases, physical structure, are risk factors that we must keep in mind when evaluating our patients, research and clinical experience continue to suggest that a person's psychosocial status and psychosocial functioning are critical in both the development of facial muscle pain and predicting responsiveness to treatment. We believe that a combination of environmental, emotional, behavioral, and physiological factors are truly at the heart of our patients' troubles. While pain symptoms may come on suddenly, the physiological processes responsible for the pain are the direct result of the brain's inability over time to maintain the normal functioning of the circulatory and neural systems that serve the muscles of the jaw, other facial areas, and neck. Years of patient care have led us to firmly believe that our muscles reflect our emotions, and that the emotional motor system described by Kurt Olsson is a true physiological reality.

Whether a person has experienced profound stress from a single event or from an ongoing source of personal distress, the end result appears to be an alteration in the brain's ability to adapt and function. Following devastating events such as rape or natural disaster, people who are suffering emotionally and psychologically are sometimes diagnosed with post-traumatic stress disorder, or PTSD. Although ongoing issues such as marital discord, relentless pressure to perform at work, or the anguish associated with a persistent medical problem may seem to be less devastating than a single traumatic event, the physical symptoms experienced by both groups likely have a common origin. The chemical and physical changes that occur in the muscles, nerves, tendons, and ligaments and result in pain are the end result of a process that begins in the brain. Until this concept is universally embraced, patients with facial pain problems will continue to come to our offices and ask, "Doctor, why does my face still ache?"

## The "Mind-Body Connection": How Emotions Cause Physical Changes in the Muscles and Result in Pain

How does this process happen, exactly? That our emotions can cause actual physical changes in our muscles that result in pain? In essence, when the brain is continually challenged by persistent emotions, its ability to regulate various bodily systems is often compromised, including the neural, circulatory, and immune systems. This compromised ability, in turn, leads to altered muscle biochemistry and the eventual emergence of pain. Ultimately, as the brain "overload" continues from the stressors of life—which often manifest as the negative emotions of anxiety and anger— the location of the pain broadens, the intensity often increases, and muscle dysfunction becomes worse. This situation is often exacerbated, in turn, by repetitive behaviors we are apt to develop unwittingly, in response to negative emotions and pain, such as clenching the teeth, bracing the jaw muscles, or elevating the shoulders, among many others. Without quick resolution of this situation, it is likely that patients' anxiety, suffering, and pain will increase, even though they have been reassured there is nothing seriously physically wrong with them.

While the brain's inability to maintain normal muscle function is the catalyst for your pain, it is important to emphasize that the pain is not "in your head." Real physical changes have occurred in muscles and their associated nerves and tissues. Once muscle physiology has been altered, the potential for symptoms of pain and mechanical difficulties increase. Though the physical changes in the muscles may be subtle with no swelling or observable findings, the pain can be severe. What are the real physical changes that occur in muscles to produce pain? This is explained immediately below.

## *"Fight or Flight," the Autonomic Nervous System, and Facial Pain*

When people experience a great deal of stress in their lives, the autonomic nervous system is often unable to fulfill its normal role of keeping our bodies functioning optimally. The autonomic nervous system controls the body's involuntary functions, such as heart rate, respiratory rate, and temperature regulation, and prepares the body for the so-called "fight or flight" reaction when a person feels threatened.

When stress or emotional upset produces the fight or flight reaction, the heart beats faster, blood pressure goes up, and blood rushes to the brain and parts of the body that need to get ready for battle. When this happens, other less critical body regions, such as the face, and associated muscles, nerves, tendons, and ligaments do not get the blood and oxygen they need to function optimally. When muscles, as well as tendons, nerves, and ligaments in the jaw, other facial areas, and neck are deprived of blood and oxygen, the individual is likely to experience symptoms that include pain, uncomfortable sensations, functional impairments, soreness, and tightness, among other symptoms.

In addition, during a fight or flight response, the body's adrenal glands produce increased levels of adrenaline and cortisol, which are hormones that, over time, can compromise immune functions and decrease both the efficiency of cellular repair and the body's ability to control inflammation.

The longer this scenario persists, patients begin to experience symptoms in other organs and areas of the body, along with their facial pain symptoms. This phenomenon is evidenced by many of our patients, who simultaneously report gastrointestinal symptoms, high blood pressure, and sleep dysfunction along with their facial pain. Research has linked, for example, facial pain of muscle origin and temporomandibular dysfunction (TMD) with Irritable Bowel Syndrome (de Leeuw, 2008). These conditions frequently co-exist because they likely share a similar origin within the autonomic nervous system. In addition, it is now known that the trigeminal nerve (which serves the jaw muscles) and the vagus nerve (which serves the stomach) are functionally intertwined, which helps to explain why jaw problems so often co-exist with the report of gastrointestinal distress when the nerves are challenged by a brain under siege.

## Reduced Blood Flow, Stress, and Facial Pain

Whether our patients have been suffering with facial pain for months or years, or have only recently been suffering, both of these patient groups experience muscle tenderness and pain conditions that seem to lack obvious tissue damage. This muscle tenderness, which is a key physical finding from examining our facial pain patients, directly results from an altered chemical environment caused by decreased blood flow through the capillary networks that serve the muscles of the face. As a result of this altered chemical environment, free nerve endings in the muscles (called metaboreceptors and nociceptors) are activated and barrage the brain with excitatory signals. Over time, sensitization and referred pain mechanisms will cause various symptoms to emerge that are associated with muscle dysfunction.

This diminished blood flow is due either to an autonomic nervous system that has begun to falter or to persistent and excessive contracture of muscles, which is brought on by learned behaviors that develop as a result of anxiety and life's daily challenges. In both cases, the end result is oxygen depletion (called hypoxia), tender muscles, and the emergence of variable symptoms (Mense, 2003). Common patient complaints include pain (sensory expression), muscle tension/contracture (motor expression), and altered sensations such as a feeling of numbness and warmth in the facial region (neural expression). These symptoms may respond to treatment quickly or linger, based on how long they have been present and whether perpetuating factors have been addressed.

## "Empty" Learned Behaviors that Create Muscle Pain

A brain under siege not only upsets the normal functioning of the autonomic nervous system, but it often causes individuals to develop various behaviors that, if repeated frequently enough, lead to muscle overutilization and the initiation and increase of painful symptoms.

Dentists, orthodontists, and facial pain doctors, among other healthcare professionals, commonly refer to such behaviors as *parafunctional* habits, or "empty" functions. They refer to the habitual exercise of a body part in a way that is other than the most common use of that body part. The list of daytime parafunctional behaviors includes bracing the jaw muscles; furrowing the brow; raising the shoulders; biting the lip, cheek, tongue, nails and cuticles; chewing gum; biting on pencils and plastic items, such as pens; and, most commonly, persistent tooth contact or clenching. These activities can fatigue both facial muscles (especially those in the jaw) and neck muscles, and create an environment of muscle tension that reduces capillary blood flow.

The most typical daytime overuse problem among patients we have treated is persistent tooth contact. As previously noted, the upper and lower teeth should never be in continuous contact. With the teeth together, you are "making a fist in your face," as if you were preparing for battle. This is a position of fight or flight, and not a posture that you can sustain without consequences. In this braced position, muscle energy is burned and fatigue develops. Muscles are caught in a vicious cycle where recovery is not possible until your jaw posture is changed.

For many of our patients, persistent tooth contact or clenching during the day is a posture that reflects an upset emotional state, or the aspiration to achieve no matter the price. Initial efforts to change this pattern are often accompanied by patients' comments such as "My face hurts more if I try to keep my teeth apart," "I have to think about keeping my teeth separated," or "Can't you just give me something to prop my jaws open?" Although considerable focus is required to eliminate this parafunctional habit, remarkable reductions in symptoms are often realized with this single behavioral change alone.

### Sleep Bruxism

Overuse of the jaw muscles also occurs during the sleeping hours as a result of what has been termed bruxism. Bruxism is derived from the Greek word *brychein,* meaning gnashing of the teeth. Biblical references such as "He teareth me in his wrath, and he gnastheth upon me with his teeth," suggest that even long ago this activity was associated with emotional states of anger, hate, fear and spirits.

Presently, bruxism has been defined as an oral parafunction (oromotor activity) characterized by grinding or clenching of the teeth during sleep, which is associated with an excessive (intense) sleep arousal state. Though grinding of the teeth gets most of the attention in discussions and advertisements, our experience suggests that night clenching is more common. In either case, the latest research suggests that these activities are prompted by activity in the brain (arousals) that prevents you from entering into the deepest parts of the sleep cycle.

Many of our patients speak of restless sleep patterns and often awaken with their face in a vice grip, with their teeth slammed together. As a result, they often report morning facial and jaw pain, which is the result of overworked and fatigued muscles from hours of contracture.

Ongoing scientific investigations (Murphy, 2008) suggest that emotional turmoil is one possible source of brain arousal during sleep. Along with tooth clenching and grinding, which may result from these arousals, research studies have identified high levels of the hormone epinephrine in the morning urine of individuals who have spent the night clenching or grinding their teeth. This finding has strengthened the notion that sleep bruxism is related to changes in the autonomic nervous system. Though there are countless individuals in this world who grind or clench their teeth at night without pain or muscular consequences, grinding and clenching—when combined with other risk factors, such as chronic psychological distress and life challenges—clearly puts the muscles of the face, jaw, and neck at risk.

### Empty Behaviors, the Neck, and Facial Pain

Approximately 40% of our patients with facial pain, including ear pain, headaches, and jaw pain—or with symptoms in their eyes or teeth—are in trouble as a result of a problem that started in their neck. These patients often cannot believe how tender their neck muscles are when examined, and they often have a difficult time embracing the reality that their facial pain has its origin in their neck. It takes a great deal of overwork, empty behaviors, stress, or emotional turmoil to fatigue these heavy-duty neck muscles.

As explained earlier, an intimate relationship exists between and among the muscles of the neck and face, the cervical nerves (which originate in the upper part of the spinal cord), the facial nerve, and the trigeminal nerve (the main nerve that transmits sensations from the face and jaw to the brain). As a result, excitation of the nerves in the neck quite often prompts the emergence of symptoms in the jaw and other areas of the face. These symptoms include pain, tension, tingling, weakness and fatigue.

Just as the jaw muscles are often contracted excessively when faced with the challenges of life, the neck muscles also are often pushed beyond their limits by the physiologic changes that accompany a brain under siege. It is not uncommon for a person who has faced persistent emotional duress to maintain a posture with their head down, a position that can be interpreted as that of resignation to a difficult set of life circumstances. In this bowed head position, the chin is lowered by lengthening the neck muscles. Since these muscles are not designed to maintain such an increased length, this overuse can lead to the typical pattern of local muscle soreness, muscle guarding, sensitization and trigger point activity. The end result is often facial pain, jaw dysfunction, or both.

## The Stages of Facial Pain from a Brain Under Siege

Facial pain that originates from a brain under siege almost always proceeds through a number of clearly identifiable stages. After reading this section, you'll understand exactly why a reduced blood flow to muscles causes them to hurt, why muscles can be functioning properly but the nerves running through them may still be firing at a heightened level leading to pain, and why your brain may interpret normal signals it receives as noxious, leading you to perceive and experience pain.

### Stage 1: Muscle Soreness

In Stage 1, as the autonomic nervous system continues to falter from a brain under siege, or as learned behaviors that result from stress fatigue the facial muscles, blood flow and oxygen levels remain diminished. The diminished oxygen level—which is needed to maintain energy in muscle tissue—changes the chemical environment in the muscle tissue, and nerve endings within the muscles and tendons become irritated. As a result, they fire more readily and lead to variable symptoms, such as sharp pain, generalized discomfort, muscle tightness and, at times, tingling or numbness.

**Anaerobic Metabolism and the Toxic "Chemical Soup."** As the oxygen level remains reduced, a process called anaerobic metabolism takes over, leading to more profound changes in the muscle biochemistry. Anaerobic metabolism essentially enables the muscles to produce energy without adequate supplies of oxygen. As a result of this process, a "chemical soup" is created that bathes the muscles, fascia, and intertwined neural tissues. This chemical soup consists of the diminished oxygen and a build-up of acidic chemicals that are harmful to the muscles and cause local muscle soreness during this first stage.

## Stage 2: Muscle Guarding

With time, this chemical soup can disrupt the key structural elements of muscle tissue: sarcomeres. The smallest functional units of muscle tissue, sarcomeres are designed to allow a muscle to contract. When the sarcomeres are immersed in this chemical soup, the muscles no longer function properly, which leads to quick fatigue and diminished movement capacity. This stage has been termed muscle splinting or guarding, and is most often responsible for the inability of our patients to open their mouths or turn their heads to a normal degree.

As a result of muscle guarding, energy reserves are continually being utilized. As energy supplies dwindle, muscles that require the same amount of energy to relax as they did to contract find it impossible to return to a normal resting posture. With time, these contracted muscles are predisposed to an even further drop in the volume of fresh blood flowing through them. The end result of this accumulation of irritating chemicals is a stage called peripheral sensitization.

## Stage 3: Peripheral Sensitization

Peripheral sensitization is typically marked by an increase in pain, sometimes to an extreme degree. Because the pain associated with peripheral sensitization can be so intense, patients assume that they have suffered a significant injury to their muscles. In fact, however, there is no injury.

The severe pain is the result of hypersensitive nerve endings within the muscles, which are now firing more readily and with more intensity. This occurs because the threshold for peripheral nerves to fire is reduced when these nerves are kept in contact with the irritating chemical soup that accompanies muscle guarding. Once peripheral nerves have become sensitized, even normal function creates pain and patients typically report pain in more locations. Patients whose symptoms begin in their face often also experience pain and sensitivity within the mouth, especially in their gums and teeth, or in their scalp, especially when they comb or wash their hair. Other individuals are afraid to put their face on a pillow or to get kissed on the cheek, as this increases their pain. Along with pain, the sensitization process may give rise to symptoms of burning and a feeling of temperature alteration in the skin of the face. As a result of the intense symptoms that accompany sensitization, many of our patients with jaw pain begin to avoid use of their jaw muscles.

This is well illustrated by a patient who came into the consultation room with a letter that began, "Technically, I am able to speak, but since my jaw seizes up after just a handful of sentences, I am writing to explain my situation in the hope that you can help me." She went on to say that she had not eaten solid foods for 5 weeks, and was living on a diet of liquids and baby foods. "The only time my jaw feels okay," she continued, "is when I first get up in the morning. After that, any movement at all, whether eating or talking, causes my face and jaw to seize up and spasm and become increasingly painful." It was clear that this woman was experiencing the effects of peripheral sensitization.

## Stage 4: Central Sensitization

When peripheral sensitization continues over time, the brain is barraged with electrical information that is perceived as pain. If the brain continues to be barraged, many of the built-in mechanisms of the central nervous system that are designed to blunt pain experiences begin to function inefficiently. As a result, the pain becomes more severe. The brain begins to interpret even *normal* incoming signals from a specific body location as pain, and the process of central sensitization is established.

**Brain Plasticity.** In this context, it is critical to remember that the brain controls muscle tone and posturing. The brain continually receives and interprets signals from specific body regions and then responds to these signals. If the response signals going back to the body from the brain persistently impact adversely on the facial muscles, then symptoms will likely emerge. In the most unfortunate situations, in response to an ongoing barrage of nerve signals, the brain's structural organization changes, as well as the way in which it processes information. This is called brain plasticity, and it can lead to chronic pain that often remains unresponsive to treatment, particularly if that treatment is directed solely at the site of the pain experience. This is exactly what happened with 53-year-old William.

William came in for a consultation because of facial pain he experienced every single day. His symptoms included persistent pain in his upper jaw on the right and left sides, particularly in the extraction sites of four molar teeth that had been removed several months earlier. He also complained of jaw tension, muscle tension in his face and head, and ear pain. William described his pain level as a 5 out of 10, and he was concerned that his personality was changing as a result.

William started his search for pain relief with his family dentist, as his first symptom was vague toothache pain in an upper left tooth. Unsure of what was wrong, his dentist sent him to a root canal specialist. As William's symptoms grew more acute and spread to the right side, first one tooth and then a second tooth were treated with root canal therapy. With no relief obtained, William consulted with a periodontist and two oral surgeons. By the time he finished his last treatment, four teeth had been extracted over a 6-month period.

What started out as a specific site of pain over an upper left tooth had become a widespread pain problem that clearly had elements of both peripheral and central sensitization. Despite the fact that four teeth were missing, William was still experiencing tooth pain. It was clear that for treatment to be successful, the focus needed to move away from the teeth and be directed at not only changing how the brain interpreted signals coming from the tooth extraction sites, but also reducing the number of signals still coming from the over-contracted and irritated muscles of his face. William's history revealed a tension-filled world of business travel and meetings that prompted both limited and disrupted sleep for weeks at a time and a learned behavior of daily tooth contact, as he attempted to manage the stress of his work obligations. Consequently, his muscles that had been at risk for years were finally pushed over the edge and tooth pain symptoms emerged.

Eventually William's pain was alleviated with understanding and treatment directed as his dysfunctional jaw and neck muscles. Medications and time were required, however, to reinvigorate his brain's natural capacity to blunt the experience of pain, and to address the peripheral and central sensitization mechanisms that had led to multiple tooth extractions and his months of suffering.

## Trigger Points and Referred Pain

At about the same time that peripheral sensitization occurs, the persistent contraction of muscles often causes the formation of muscle trigger points. As previously described, trigger points are highly sensitive spots in a skeletal muscle that can give rise to pain or tenderness in another location in the body. This type of pain, as you've already learned, is called referred pain or referred tenderness. As a result of active trigger points, the location of symptoms may not represent the actual origin of the problem.

## Summary

A brain under siege by emotions from life challenges can no longer attend to its normal, daily obligations in an efficient way. Emotional turmoil disrupts the way the autonomic nervous system operates. As a result, homeostasis is lost in terms of controlling blood flow to muscles, regulating nerve discharge, and maintaining normal muscle tone. As blood flow drops off, so does the level of oxygen brought to the muscles. Less oxygen means more potential for anaerobic metabolism and the buildup of nasty chemicals, such as lactic acid, which are irritating to nerves.

This altered chemical environment not only leads to muscle soreness and pain, but also to physical changes in the muscles. Such physical changes lead, in turn, to the formation of trigger points that can refer pain, along with muscle weakness and contracture.

As muscle performance is compromised, symptoms become more debilitating and of concern to the now anxious patient. In addition, the altered chemical environment of the muscles predisposes the nerve endings in the muscle tissues to fire at a lower threshold. Consequently, even normal stimuli can now produce pain, an occurrence called sensitization.

As a result of this entire process, which represents a psychophysiologic problem, the brain essentially sets the muscles up for failure, and anguish alone can disrupt the brain's ability to serve muscles adequately.

Furthermore, a brain under siege by emotions from life challenges and uncontrollable circumstances will prompt people to develop or learn "empty" behaviors that involve the jaw, other facial muscles (especially those used for facial expression), the neck and the shoulders. These empty behaviors may be limited to certain situations, prompting the emergence of symptoms only when the patient is, for example, working or studying, or they may become part of the patient's normal posture in all environments. In fact, changing these abnormal muscle tendencies feels strange to patients after awhile.

Many of these learned behaviors, such as tooth contact during the day, furrowing the brow, jutting the jaw, and pernicious nail and cuticle biting, take muscles that are normally designed to be sprinters and turn them into long distance runners. In addition, smiling all day to help prompt sales or frowning as a result of emotional distress can also tax muscles.

As a result, the sprinting muscles, which are acting like long distance runners, fatigue and falter in performance, with the same adverse effects as previously discussed. Over time the persistence of these empty, learned behaviors or tendencies exceed the threshold for these muscles to cope and, as a result, they ache and the cycle begins.

If the patient doesn't understand that these learned behaviors are potentially destructive, the cycle continues and the pain persists. With time, the field of pain spreads and involves innocent structures, such as the teeth, ears, and sinuses, which drive the patient to seek professional care and go from office to office, in search of an answer that is elusive.

Figure 10 on the next page depicts the somewhat complex interrelationship between the factors discussed in this chapter—including emotions, a brain under siege, muscle pain, and empty, learned behaviors.

Figure 10: Interrelationship between Emotions, a Brain Under Siege, Muscle Pain, and Empty, Learned Behaviors

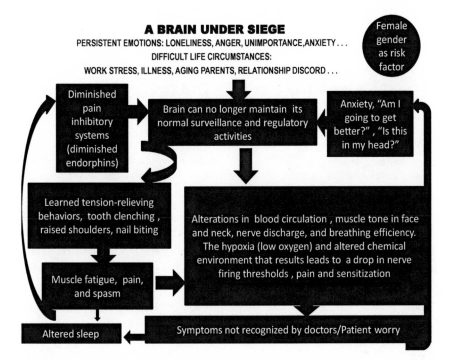

## Chapter 6

# GETTING THE PROPER DIAGNOSIS AND TREATMENT FOR PERSISTENT FACIAL PAIN

*Some patients, though conscious that their condition is perilous, recover their health simply through their contentment with the goodness of the physician.* — Hippocrates

From the preceding chapter, you now understand that most persistent facial pain is usually the result of muscles that have been chemically and structurally altered by a brain under siege. The majority of patients with facial pain do not know this, however, and so their first impulse is to see a dentist, ENT specialist, neurologist, or other healthcare professional, based on their learned experience and the location of their troublesome symptoms. Eventually, however, some of these patients either see a facial pain doctor on their own or are referred to one by their dentist or physician, after failing to get the relief they were seeking.

The first thing these patients want to know, of course, is how and when they are going to feel better. As you might expect, the answer will vary from person to person, based on the circumstances that have led to their muscle pain, how long they have been in trouble, and whether or not treatment along the way has complicated their problem.

### What We Do First: Validating Patients' Symptoms

One of our primary goals is to validate your symptoms and make sure you understand that your pain is real and has a legitimate source. Although you may have seen multiple doctors and undergone numerous treatments without benefit, you should not assume you are "crazy" and that your pain is "in your mind."

Depending on the stage of muscle dysfunction, patients may get relief just by knowing we understand their problem and have successfully treated it in the past. As part of the first visit, patients learn their problem is common, and that there is no reason why they cannot be helped. Often, just being told there is light at the end of the tunnel reduces patients' pain and/or suffering, particularly if they are frustrated from trying to get medical help over and over again without success.

Although we may communicate confidence that we can relieve your pain, we never use the word "cure," which is more appropriate for patients with a disease, injury, or who are sick. Our goal is to identify why your muscles are malfunctioning and reduce or eliminate your pain. Our treatment strategies are designed to diminish the severity, duration, and intensity of your symptoms, and give nature a chance to promote healing in both mind and body. By setting realistic goals for symptom reduction, your painful muscles can recover in stages—first, 25% less pain, then 50% less pain, then more if treatment is going well.

Once patients become aware of the reasons their muscles are in trouble, we can work on reducing their symptoms and eliminating their impact on daily activities, while simultaneously decreasing medication use, inspiring optimism, and instructing patients on how to prevent new episodes of suffering. Most patients improve markedly once they understand that they do not have an underlying disease or injury to prevent them from getting better, and they make the connection between their daily life and their brain's impaired capacity to maintain muscle comfort. The case of Hillary provides an excellent example of how awareness of the mind-body connection can result in the cessation of pain.

When Hillary, an attractive 45-year-old woman, first came to the office, she was well-dressed and appeared to be a confident person, in control of her world and comfortable in her own skin. Her only problem seemed to be that she complained of throbbing, persistent headaches in her temples that were so painful they interfered with her normal daily activities. She had previously seen a number of doctors and dentists who put her through medical testing that had not provided any answers. Her headaches were not caused by vascular or neurological problems, weather changes, alcohol, or food allergies. All of the possible organic origins for this pain had been ruled out. Our examination, however, revealed that the muscles in her temples were extremely tender. Further questioning and

71

examination did not reveal the presence of learned behaviors that could be responsible for the reactive state of these muscles. Why, then, did Hillary's muscles hurt so much, and were they at the root of her headache pain?

While speaking with Hillary about her life—in an attempt to uncover possible personal issues that might be at the root of her chronic pain—she revealed the source of her problem. Hillary had been married for 20 years and didn't have any children. Her husband was one of several brothers who managed a string of very successful retail stores, and he was busy working much of the time during the week. To maintain tight control of his complex business operation, Hillary's husband and his brothers met every Friday night for dinner and business planning. The spouses were never invited to these meetings, which lasted well into the night.

Also on Friday nights special dinners were held at the country club to which Hillary and her husband belonged. These dinners were popular social events attended by many of Hillary's friends and their husbands, but Hillary was not comfortable going alone, so she stayed at home by herself. On Saturdays the country club hosted golf and dining events that again brought together club members. Hillary's husband, tired from the week's work, would not attend, and Hillary once again would not go alone. For Hillary's husband, spending time with her and socializing with their friends was not a priority. It was clear that Hillary's loneliness, anger, and resentment created an emotional state that produced her chronic headaches.

For Hillary the resolution was simple. Once she understood and became aware of her emotional state, she began to go to the club without her husband and, as anticipated, he soon started coming home early enough on Friday nights to be with her. On Saturday nights, he was awake enough to participate in the club's activities. As if by magic, Hillary's headaches disappeared.

Hillary's story clearly represents the reality that thoughts and feelings alone (resentment of being left out, loneliness, anger) are sufficient to drive the experience of pain. Hillary's symptoms were a *cri de coeur*, a cry from the heart. We believe that the anger, resentment, and dismay she felt from being kept out of the world she wanted to be a part of created an emotional state that manifested itself as a physical complaint: "I have a headache."

When patients present with this kind of scenario, which unfortunately is rather frequent, where the level of suffering is high but the physical evidence for the complaints is low, our role is to assure them that their symptoms are no less real than if they occurred from a physical trauma. At the same time, we try to make such patients aware that the resolution of their symptoms will only follow the resolution of their personal conflicts. From time to time, we have found it necessary to recommend patients for psychosocial evaluations, although many of them often reject this suggestion. As one patient said, "I will not go down that path. Too many of my friends ended up divorced after therapy."

Though Hillary's pain experience was driven by thoughts alone, our experience has made it clear that it is more common for a cumulative combination of risk factors to push patients "over the edge," and their symptoms follow. Most of the time, the management or elimination of a few emotionally-driven risk factors seems to be sufficient, and symptoms improve markedly or disappear. Joan is just one example of how this works.

When 45-year-old Joan came to our office, she described persistent left facial pain, swelling on the left side of her face, and years of intermittent tooth pains, which had prompted several episodes of root canal therapy and a number of surgical procedures that never fully stopped her suffering. Past medical evaluations had never uncovered a reason for her facial pain, and dental interventions that were performed to address her symptoms were ultimately unsuccessful.

Joan clearly had a life full of past and present emotional turmoil, and she lived in the world with her teeth constantly touching. This behavioral tendency developed as she faced daily life challenges. Joan was in essence "making a fist in her face" on a daily basis, compromising muscles and leading to the variety and severity of symptoms that she had experienced over several years. Once Joan learned to keep her teeth from touching during the day, her pain and symptoms were reduced significantly. Though her life circumstances had not changed, the elimination of a significant risk factor resulted in a major reduction of her symptoms.

## Patient Participation in the Treatment Process: The 60/40 Rule

We believe that patients must actively participate in the treatment process if they want to get better, rather than simply being a passive recipient of our efforts. It is only when both doctor and patient accept an active role that long-term healing can occur. We have come to call this doctor-patient collaboration the 60/40 rule. At times, the patient contributes 60% to his or her own treatment and the doctor contributes 40%, or vice versa, based on the stage of muscle compromise. In other words, most of the patients we see do not have "Doctor, fix me!" problems, as mentioned earlier, but, rather, problems that require patient responsibility to implement the plan of treatment.

The goal of this philosophy and approach is both to empower patients, so they can take credit for their immediate improvement, and give them the skills necessary to prevent setbacks in the future. Whether the treatment requires changing behaviors, taking medication, performing exercises at home, participating in counseling, or regularly doing simple breathing or relaxation techniques, our patients are continually told that healing is a process that will require time and their full participation. Patient ownership of the healing process is second only to our validation of their problem. When we achieve improved resiliency of mind and muscle, our goals have been realized.

## The Importance of Listening to Patients with Facial Pain

A wise colleague of ours once said, "Never treat a stranger." These simple words are one of the keys to understanding chronic facial pain. Getting to know our patients can be critical to successful treatment. When we meet a patient for the first time, we begin by saying, "What troubles you?" From there, we follow an approach explained so well by the noted physician Sir William Osler in his best known saying: "Listen to your patient, he is telling you the diagnosis" (Osler Symposia, 2011). This adage, which emphasizes the importance of taking a good history, we might paraphrase as saying: "The diagnosis is in the history if we choose to listen, but most of us are deaf." Listening is especially important since patients sometimes describe their symptoms in a way that can lead us down a wrong path, when we are trying to identify what is causing them to have facial pain.

In today's medical world, most doctors don't have the time to listen and, as a result, they often miss the most critical clues to the origin of a patient's pain. Encouraging patients to talk and listening carefully to their stories have proven to be powerful diagnostic tools.

Though just listening to a patient doesn't always give rise to an accurate diagnosis, careful listening can often provide important insights into the nature of the problem and help rule out conditions that probably don't exist. The case of Patricia, 52 years old, shows how conversation can be a critical part of an examination.

Patricia arrived at the office wearing dark sunglasses on a cold, wet February morning. As she talked and took off the glasses, it was obvious she had a condition called proptosis, which causes bulging of the eyes and is presumed to result from a thyroid disease. As she described the problem that brought her to the office, it was clear that her story was similar to so many other women with her type of pain. She had pain in her jaw when she opened her mouth and pain in her temples. The most interesting and revealing part of what she said occurred when we asked her if there was a specific time of day she was in pain or if the pain was constant throughout the day. She said that in the morning the pain was minimal or non-existent and that it peaked each day at about 4 p.m., but she wasn't sure why.

In the course of this first visit, she also said she had been under treatment for a thyroid gland deficiency, but that it was not a problem for her. Later in the visit, however, she said there had been two unsuccessful surgical efforts to correct the problem.

When the visit was over, Patricia had provided enough information to allow for a diagnosis of her pain, at least partially, but it seemed unusual that the pain would peak at exactly 4 p.m. each day, which suggested that a piece of the puzzle was missing.

On her second visit, Patricia was more at ease and she offered a possible source of the 4 p.m. onset of pain. She said that her husband expected dinner to be on the table at exactly 6 p.m. every evening when he came home from work, and Patricia found this rigidity very difficult to handle. She asked if that could actually be the reason for her pain, which led to a discussion about the important role anxiety and tension can often play in the genesis of physiological changes that can produce pain. It was suggested that the stress in her life might be the root of her problem, since she had no detectable disease or injury.

Two weeks later, Patricia came in for her third visit, and by this time she felt she could be open and honest about her feelings. When asked if there was anything she wished to add, she said that as a result of her two visits, she came to realize that the two elements of her life that caused the most tension—her bulging eyes and her husband's demands—were causing her facial pain. She declared that neither of these factors should have the power to exert such a negative impact on how she functioned, and scheduled an appointment in 1 month for a follow-up.

At that time Patricia reported that her headaches and jaw pain were gone. Understanding the root of her pain, getting validation of her symptoms and concerns during the treatment process, and confronting her problem head-on were all that needed to be done. As it turned out, Patricia's husband didn't care that dinner wasn't always ready exactly on time every night, and Patricia realized that much of the pressure she had felt had been self-imposed.

## Persistent and Multiple Symptoms

Many of our patients over the years with persistent systems have been trapped in a cycle of pain and dysfunction. We consider it important to know about persistent symptoms in the facial area and in other parts of the body to be able to best diagnose and treat our patients. Based on our experience and research, we have identified four common factors that allow us to predict symptom persistence in our facial pain patients:

1. They report pain in other parts of the body along with their facial pain.

2. They have a significant number of painful sites in the facial and cervical, or upper neck, region.

3. They complain about frequent pain every day.

4. They have problems with other organ systems along with their facial pain, such as irritable bowel syndrome (IBS), gastroesophageal reflux disease (GERD), chronic fatigue syndrome, hypertension, dermatitis, insomnia, depression, and anxiety.

These characteristics help alert us to challenges we may face as we attempt to relieve a patient's facial pain. With the knowledge that we have only five or six common treatment options, it is important to establish expectations before we put treatment in place. For a patient with one or more of the above characteristics, it is likely that, even if we make substantial progress, the time frame to achieve that progress and the ability to maintain it will be unpredictable.

For patients with frequent pain in multiple locations, it is likely that both peripheral and central sensitization mechanisms are driving the symptoms (see Chapter 5). Because these influences are so powerful, we consider it crucial to define treatment goals at the outset—such as pain reduction, less use of over-the-counter medications, and/or increased eating ability—to help patients avoid ongoing disappointment and worry, which can contribute to their continued pain.

The presence of other problems in our facial pain patients, such as IBS, GERD, and chronic fatigue syndrome, to name only a few, is not a surprising or new finding. Years ago, writings in the dental literature posited that if a brain under siege is able to disrupt normal muscle function and physiology, then it makes sense that additional broad-based symptoms in other organ regions will emerge—and they will likely be due to the same sensitization mechanisms that produce the primary symptoms of facial pain. The presence of multiple organ systems in trouble at the same time is clear evidence of a brain under siege, as may be seen in the case of Molly.

Sixteen-year-old Molly, a high school junior, came for treatment with her mother trailing right behind her. They were a matched pair as reflected in their dress, posture, and voice—except that Molly was in pain. Prior to a physical examination, a conversation with Molly revealed that she was a high-achieving, very busy young girl, an "A" student who sang in her school's chorus and played flute in the orchestra. She was planning to go on a European tour with the school orchestra, but her facial pain had put that plan temporarily on hold.

Articulate and sensitive, Molly was under constant pressure to do well academically and musically. Not only did she have high expectations for herself, but her mom also set the bar very high. Molly was clearly anxious, and her facial muscles—used to sing and play the flute—were paying the price. As an unconscious response to the stress in her life, Molly clenched her teeth off and on all day, and the tension had caused her muscles to tighten and shorten, resulting in facial pain. The pain started off as episodic and moderate in intensity, but had become constant and severe. When she came to our office she could barely open her mouth.

Of even more concern was that Molly had been diagnosed with irritable bowel syndrome, and her chronic eczema had gotten worse. For such a young girl, she was experiencing three physical manifestations of persistent emotional stress: IBS, eczema, and the fatigue and contracture of her jaw muscles. Molly and her parents had ignored the alarm bell that first sounded in her stomach and then in her skin.

Though her facial pain and muscle spasms eased with treatment within a short period of time, Molly and her parents needed to take a careful look at her world and make whatever changes were necessary to get her brain out of a state of siege. If ignored, Molly's future would likely be full of physical ailments that would impact the quality of her life. From experience with many adult patients who have had facial pain accompanied by other ailments, including fibromyalgia, GERD, chronic fatigue syndrome, insomnia and Epstein-Barr virus, Molly's future was not difficult to predict.

In treatment, Molly was continually reassured that although her facial pain was severe, it was not due to a terrible disease and that she would get better in time. The focus of her treatment was based on the concept that her problems were not started by a single event or activity, but, rather, were due to a number of risk factors that rendered her brain incapable of maintaining control over her muscles, skin, and stomach functions. The conversation, insight, and support Molly got in treatment were critical components of her care. Most importantly, Molly recognized that she had to own her problem and take full responsibility for either the success or failure of treatment. The 60/40 rule certainly applied in her case, with Molly ultimately doing the majority of the work.

## Three Common Patient Profile Groups

We have categorized our patients into three general groups. While each group suffers from facial pain that begins in the brain, their profiles are quite different. An upset brain can give rise to physiological changes at different severity levels based on many factors. For some patients recovery is easy, while for others it is more difficult. Depending on the profile group a patient is in, the treatment strategy differs. More specifically, within each group of patients treatment strategies are based on two factors: (1) the stage of their muscle pain and malfunction and (2) the circum-stances that prompted the onset of their problem. The strategies are focused on the process of symptom reduction and designed to confront the factors that have overwhelmed the brain's ability to regulate muscle tone, posture, and function.

## Group 1: Patients with Pain as a Result of Everyday Challenges

Patients in Group 1 are the most common. They experience facial pain because of ordinary, everyday challenges, such as raising children, supporting a family, achieving in school, running a successful business, and dealing with the central responsibilities of life. Due to the stress they experience, they often develop behaviors such as biting their nails, clenching their teeth, chewing on pens, or raising their shoulders habitually. Their muscles become overused and overworked, as a result, which eventually leads to muscle fatigue and pain. Dom, who had intense facial pain during the week but not on the weekends, was a classic example of this type of patient.

Thirty-five-year-old Dom was outgoing and friendly, but it was obvious that he was in a lot of pain. Though he awakened in the morning without pain, within a few hours jaw and facial pain would come on predictably, and he experienced difficulty opening his mouth. Most revealing was that this only occurred Monday through Friday. Those were the days he drove a truck that delivered cement to construction sites all over New York City on a strict time schedule. Dom was aware that he had to arrive at the sites before the cement hardened. To do this, he had to negotiate the crowded streets and intersections of Manhattan at the busiest times of day, and then had to back his truck up to specific locations on the sites so he could unload the cement. This created a great deal of stress for him. His jaw pain added to the stress and made him even more anxious.

In questioning Dom further about his routine, including small details that might not have seemed important initially, he laughed and said that as soon as he started up his truck, he put an unlit cigar in his mouth and bit down on that cigar all day long. At this point, Dom simply thought of it as a harmless habit that, at first, helped to relieve stress. At night, Dom was calm, didn't have a cigar in his mouth, and was pain-free. What Dom didn't consider was that biting down on a cigar all day to relieve tension was overloading the muscles that open and close the jaw. These muscles finally went into contraction and spasm, and Dom was in severe pain.

Dom became aware of what was causing his pain and he got rid of the cigars. His pain went away and he listened to music instead, to help alleviate the tension created by his job. Dom was in a never-ending cycle that began with stress, but ended with pain as a result of a seemingly benign tendency. Until he learned what was going on, Dom couldn't break the cycle and get to the root of his problem.

In the course of living their busy, scheduled, and committed lives, patients in this first profile group exhaust their facial and/or neck muscles. Their brain, which is continually aroused by life circumstances and decisions, sets the stage for problems to develop. As muscles cannot remain in a contracted and tense state, symptoms inevitably emerge.

The people who fall into this group have relatively simple problems that can be resolved with education, self regulation techniques, and exercises. At times, the factors "fueling the fire" of their stress and adverse behaviors drop off, such as the end of a school term or busy work project, admittance to college, or resolution of a financial problem or acute medical condition. Cessation of the stressful situation eliminates the reason the person's brain was in an excited state in the first place. When conversation and education help patients to recognize that their emotional state or life circumstance prompted a persistent behavioral pattern leading to muscle contraction, it is not uncommon for them to feel better after just a few sessions of treatment.

## Group 2: Patients with Pain as a Result of a Brain Under Siege

While patients in Group 2 also experience facial pain because of muscle problems, their muscles are not only overloaded by stress-induced activities but also compromised by a brain under siege. These people are dealing with life issues of a more serious and chronic nature over which they feel they have little or no control—such as a very sick child, a parent with Alzheimer's disease, spousal abuse, job loss, divorce, the death of a loved one, ongoing medical problems, and so on.

Many such patients arrive at the office with the knowledge that their lives are stressful and challenging, but with no insight into how these factors have given rise to their stubborn pain problems. They do not want to wear their emotions on their sleeves, so they come in with a cheerful attitude and smiling face, only to be suffering underneath it all. The pain they are experiencing is quite obviously real, but the origins remain a mystery to them. Jeanette is a typical example of a patient who wasn't making the connection between her life and her stress.

Jeannette, 38 years old, had been suffering with symptoms of facial and jaw pain for a year and a half. She had consulted with multiple doctors and had undergone various treatments without any benefit. Jeannette's medical history was unremarkable, and when she was asked about her daily life, she did not mention any turmoil or concern that might be contributing to her pain. Not surprisingly, an examination revealed a number of sore and tender jaw and neck muscles. When her neck muscles were touched, she quickly withdrew and said, "I never knew those muscles were so painful. Nobody ever examined them before."

Very little was identified in Jeannette's personal history that could be responsible for these findings. As a result, it was puzzling why she was in such trouble. As the session was about to end, Jeannette said, "Can I mention a few additional things?" At this point, she decided to share that not only had she been struggling with infertility for the last 6 years, but she had also been participating in an anger management program for the better part of 1 year. In fact, her symptoms started approximately 2 weeks after the latest medical efforts to assist her pregnancy hopes failed.

By sharing these critical pieces of information, Jeanette provided the groundwork for insights that would help her get better. Knowing that Jeanette's world was a source of emotional pain led to the conclusion that her upset brain had set the stage for her muscle pain. The goal then became clear. Treatment had to start with education so that Jeanette could understand, embrace, and identify with the reality that a brain under siege was fully capable of driving the physical and chemical changes in muscles that are responsible for the experience of facial pain. By no means did this treatment solve her infertility issues, of course, or hasten her ability to manage anger, but her newly-gained knowledge validated her suffering and provided hope that redirected treatment strategies could diminish her pain to a considerable degree.

By making a number of critical mind-body connections for Jeanette, she gained confidence that she was in control of her own destiny and would not have to live with pain, as many doctors had told her along the way. Prior to our conversations, it had never occurred to Jeanette that her persistent anger ("for the hand that I was dealt") might be responsible for her facial pain. With this knowledge, she was not only able to participate in the treatment process, but she made the critical decision to stop looking for a doctor to "fix my pain problem."

Jeanette's story is a familiar one, shared by so many patients who are not yet capable of fully appreciating how difficult life circumstances, challenges, and burdens can impact the brain to such a profound extent that pain symptoms emerge.

Patients in this group have problems that begin in the brain but are ultimately expressed in the muscles of the face (often the jaw) and the neck. They often have pain, but it is not uncommon to hear these patients complain that they also have muscle weakness and symptoms such as burning and tingling sensations in the face. These symptoms are confusing to patients and often cause them to experience increased stress. Even more confusing for patients is that the pain location may have nothing to do with its origin, due to active pain referral mechanisms (see Chapter 2).

By the time such patients arrive for treatment, their muscle problems usually have progressed to the point where conversation, validation, and education alone—though still critical—will fail to restore comfort and health in the muscle groups involved. For these patients, treatments that deal with both the compromised muscles and the psychosocial, emotional, and life factors challenging the brain are all part of the process of recovery.

For many patients with a brain under siege, once their complaints are validated, treatment starts with one or multiple therapies to reduce pain and restore optimism and control. Though these treatments are essentially directed at the end result (the muscles) of a problem that started in the brain, they are helpful in reducing suffering and allowing patients to realize that they can be helped. The most common treatments we use to get muscles on the path to recovery include behavioral self-regulation instruction (such as keeping the teeth apart), medications, various forms of physiotherapy, muscle needling techniques, nerve blocks, and a variety of oral appliances.

In addition to these treatments, conversation allows us to introduce cognitive strategies designed to assist our patients in better managing the life forces that put their muscles at risk. While many circumstances are unchangeable and personality tendencies are difficult to modify, our patients tend to improve once they better grasp the mind-body connections responsible for the muscle changes that drive their pain. A combination of self-regulation techniques and professional counseling strategies designed to quiet the mind, blended with treatments designed to physically assist muscle recovery, achieve lasting results.

The efficacy of this approach can be seen in the case of Jane, whom you first met in Chapter 4. There she described the multiple, painful symptoms she was suffering from, and her initial, frustrating attempt at finding relief through a traditional solution, which included seeing dentists, ENT specialists, and neurologists, all to no avail. Finally, she said, "I mentioned my problem to a friend who suggested that I see a dentist who was a facial pain doctor." She then went on to describe what ensued, in her own words: "When we met for the first time, Dr. Tanenbaum and I talked about what I had been through. He said that feeling better would be a process. He suspected that the pain in my teeth and face had a muscle origin and that the muscles were in trouble due to difficult life challenges and an upset brain. I'd be lying if I said that made sense to me at first. After all, although I had stress in my life, I truly thought that I was managing it well. I had always been a type-A personality, so I was used to putting lots of pressure on myself and being in control.

"Along with a number of self-regulation techniques to relax my facial muscles and a regimen of trigger point injections and physical therapy, Dr. Tanenbaum suggested that I see a psychiatrist or psycho-pharmacologist to deal with, as he put it, 'what's going on in my brain.' I definitely didn't believe that was the answer, but I was willing to do anything to get better. When I thought about the most well-known symptoms of anxiety, I thought about panic attacks, migraines, headaches—not pain in the mouth and face. I didn't know it at the time, but this was the turning point for me.

"I began treatment with a psychiatrist I knew well and trusted, and started taking an anti-anxiety medication. In a matter of weeks, I began to understand more about the causes of my anxiety and I was feeling better. I felt in control of my life again. Once I understood that the source of my mouth/facial pain was anxiety, the other treatments that had been recommended began to be much more effective. The combination of psychotherapy, medication, physical therapy, and trigger point injections gave me my life back. Each week, I felt better and better! It was clear that the anxiety that ultimately led to the mouth/facial pain didn't happen overnight, but rather built up over time.

"Today, I feel so much better. It took 9 long months, but I am enjoying life again, going out with friends regularly, and most importantly, I'm there for my daughter every day. It's the most wonderful feeling in the world. However, if you would have told me that first day when I woke up with pain on the upper left side of my mouth that the cause was anxiety, I would have never believed it, and I don't think my dentist or the many other doctors I saw would have either."

Though Jane required professional intervention to speed her path to recovery, many patients in this second category can get better without either formal counseling or medication to quiet the mind. At the outset, it is difficult to determine who will need or embrace this type of assistance. Since patients often feel threatened by the referral for counseling, or they only poorly understand it, we often wait to build trust before we encourage this aspect of care. When we are able to knit together all the necessary components of care, the pain and suffering is often reduced or eliminated.

**Teenage Patients in Patient Profile Group 2.** When young children and teens have persistent facial pain, their histories almost always point to life events and circumstances as the driving forces behind their symptoms. Over the last 10 years, more of these young patients have sought treatment for facial pain.

Even the youngest patients need to understand the connection between their life, their brain, and their pain before they can get better. This was the case with Valerie, a 13-year-old girl who came to the office after 3 days of severe pain, which she described as a "facial headache." Valerie's pediatrician and dentist both suggested that she had a jaw-related problem. It was immediately obvious from Valerie's facial expression that she was in severe pain. During examination she could hardly move her jaw, and the muscles in her jaw, other facial areas, upper shoulder, and neck region were very sensitive to the touch. Most revealing, however, was the size of her jaw muscles. When she brought her teeth together, her jaw muscles bulged visibly, revealing size and strength that could only have been generated by frequent clenching and tooth contact. In fact, at only 13 years old, Valerie had developed a tendency typically found in more mature adult patients. When faced with daily life situations, obligations, tasks, and challenges, she brought her teeth together and clenched. What was driving this destructive tendency?

In conversations with Valerie, she eventually revealed that she had a routine filled with private school rigor, self-imposed expectations, and private fencing lessons and competitions, which undoubtedly absorbed all of her time. Even her weekends were full of scheduled activities and study obligations. From this information, it became clear that she had too much to handle for a young girl, and her brain was on "overload." Her pain was like an alarm bell, signaling a problem that needed attention. As she continued to constantly clench her teeth as a response to her overloaded world and expectations of achievement, her muscle dysfunction became more and more advanced, and she ended up in severe pain.

When this was explained to her in a very simple way, she clearly understood what was going on. These insights were the first step in the process of Valerie getting better.

**ADHD and Facial Pain.** Over the last several years, we've seen an increase in both high school and college students seeking treatment of facial pain, with the typical descriptions except for one element of their history that is quite different from most patients. They were not only experiencing muscle pain as a result of the stress of academic challenges, but also were in trouble from taking medications such as Adderall, Ritalin, and Concerta for attention deficit hyperactivity disorder. These medications sometimes help focus the patient's mind and attention in order to achieve, but their use often comes with a price. Because these medications are central nervous system stimulants, muscles often react by tightening, with pain symptoms being the end result.

Since the need to achieve is so often reinforced in today's society, we anticipate that more and more patients will be seen with the unintended complication of facial pain from taking these medications, which are designed to foster increased attention, performance, and achievement.

**Facial Pain and Seniors.** On the other extreme, as our population ages, it is easy to understand why our elderly patients are suffering from symptoms of facial pain. Once medical problems and local disease have been ruled out as the source of pain, muscles must be considered. Seniors are far from being immune to the phenomenon of facial muscle pain, and there are greater concerns as life expectancy increases. Financial resources may dwindle and loneliness becomes common as spouses and friends pass away or relocate to be closer to their own children. In addition, medical infirmities may limit independence and reduce the pleasures of life. These factors, coupled with an aging musculoskeletal system, put seniors at high risk for facial muscle problems.

## Group 3: Patients with Pain but No Muscle Dysfunction

The patients in Group 3 describe their pain similarly to patients in the first two groups, but their physical examination reveals little, if any, evidence of muscle soreness or dysfunction. In these patients, where there are lots of symptoms but no detectable tissue change, we must focus more on the person and his or her specific life circumstances.

We explain to such patients that, while their experience of pain is real, it is caused not by a physical problem but, rather, by their belief that something is wrong. Furthermore, we go on to explain that while their symptoms may prompt them to go on a time-consuming search for a conventional answer, their symptoms also provide them with an opportunity to avoid facing more difficult realities.

Thirty-eight-year-old Julie is one example of a patient who falls into this category. Her visit was another attempt at getting medical help for the persistent facial pain she had experienced for 2 years. For someone who had been suffering for such a long time, her demeanor was calm, and she could not describe any specific factors that would increase her pain or alleviate suffering, even for a short period of time. It seemed right from the start that, for Julie, there were personal issues at play.

When asked about her family, Julie immediately began to speak about her two daughters, who were 4 years apart. The older daughter, Sarah, was a developmentally disabled teenager with limited learning ability. The younger daughter, Barbara, was just entering the lively and challenging life of a typical teenager. Barbara had an active social life and her friends and classmates were in and out of the house all the time. In addition, Barbara had become moody and more difficult to get along with, as is the case with many teenagers. Julie had always been anxious about taking care of Sarah and tending to her needs, but now she was also stressed about Barbara's behavior and the interaction between Sarah and Barbara's friends. It was no coincidence that, after 2 years of suffering, Julie chose now as the time to seek help.

By the end of her initial visit, it was clear that Julie's pain was not the primary issue. She needed to develop an acceptable strategy for dealing with the needs of her first-born and the evolving needs of her second child. Her pain had served a purpose. For 2 years she sought care for her facial pain, thus avoiding the more emotionally-charged need to address the difficult life realities that were surfacing at home.

Unlike patients in the first two groups, who respond to physically-based muscle therapy, Julie's physical examination revealed an absence of clearly defined muscle pain. This was the key to understanding that we could not provide the relief she had hoped to find.

## Pain and Suffering

Though Julie reported pain, she was really suffering. As briefly discussed earlier, although pain and suffering are often used interchangeably, an important distinction needs to be made. Pain is an unpleasant signal telling you that something is wrong with your body. Suffering results from the meaning or interpretation your brain assigns to the pain signal. Suffering, then, is an emotional/psychological condition, often experienced by individuals whose brains are overwhelmed by fear, anxiety, depression, hopelessness, and dread. For Julie, relief was found only after months of professional counseling and the implementation of life strategies that eased the daily challenges at home.

## A High Rate of Successful Treatment Outcomes

Since the vast majority of patients we have seen fall into the first and second groups, our success rates have been high with the strategies we employ. For the patients in the first group—whose pain is caused by overused and fatigued muscles due to stress-induced behaviors—treatment benefits are often achieved within weeks. Benefit is most often measured by a decrease in pain intensity and frequency and less need for medication. At times, education combined with the elimination of overuse tendencies, such as resting the teeth together during the day or nail biting, can quickly relieve facial pain symptoms that have been present for months or even years. It is not uncommon for patients to report, several weeks following their initial visit, that their pain has diminished to a significant degree, solely as a result of changing longstanding habits. With optimism, along with self-regulation techniques and exercises designed to restore health to the compromised muscles, further improvement occurs.

## Treating Patients with Recurring Facial Pain

Strictly speaking, most persistent facial pain problems cannot be "cured," since they are not due to disease, injury, or structural malfunction, as discussed throughout the book. The pain symptoms, which are of muscle origin, can certainly resurface, therefore, even after many years. In the presence of difficult life circumstances or in the pursuit of achievement, the brain's control over blood circulation, nerve discharge, respiratory regulation, and refreshing sleep can falter, with the end result being the re-emergence of muscle pain in the face.

Among patients who were able to get better in the past, we have found that some have relatively little difficulty recovering the second time around, due to the insights they learned about the mind-body connection, while others have more difficulty, as a result of life events that make their recovery less predictable.

The latter type of patient is illustrated by the case of Ann, who was 60 years old when she first came for treatment. Her problem, she said, was pain on the right side of her face. She explained that there was stress at home, which brought to mind the connection between her pain, her brain, and her life conditions at home. An examination clearly revealed that Ann's facial pain was referred from her neck, which prompted a few muscle trigger point injections. Not only did Ann experience an immediate decrease in her symptoms, but she seemed relieved and less anxious when she learned how stress could very well be the catalyst for her pain. On follow-up after her one visit, it was found that Ann's pain had lessened considerably, and by doing a number of exercises at home she felt considerably better.

About 7 years later, Ann returned for treatment when she began to hurt again, this time on both sides of her face, not just the right side. An examination revealed pain and muscle sensitivity in her face and temples, along with the neck and shoulders. Ann mentioned several times that her pain had been present for several months, but she delayed coming for an examination to avoid paying a fee beyond her fixed budget.

After discussing how hard it was for people today to make ends meet, particularly those in their retirement years, Ann said she was very concerned about her ex-husband's lateness with his monthly alimony payments. Apparently, the stress of worrying about receiving these payments was becoming overwhelming for her. After a few minutes of sharing her fears, Ann said, "Why am I telling you this? You are a dentist."

In the absence of underlying medical problems, it was likely that the re-emergence of Ann's symptoms had a muscular origin, because of her

88

ongoing fear that her former husband would be unpredictable in paying her alimony benefits. Loss of control and fear are common driving forces in facial pain patients, and they were playing a significant role in Ann's case.

Her treatment consisted of validating her complaint, making the connection between her life conditions and her pain, treating her with injections, and reviewing the exercises that she had found helpful in the past. Predictably, her symptoms eased, but it was likely that if her husband missed payments, her symptoms would continue. The treatment provided bought Ann some time, prevented her muscle dysfunction from reaching the next level, and provided reassurance that nothing was terribly wrong. At times, this is the best that facial pain doctors can do.

Unlike Ann and patients like her, many other patients who return for care have much more predictable and positive outcomes. Their stories provide a great deal of insight into the true origins of facial pain problems. John's case provides a good example of this type of patient, and his story makes it clear why we believe emotions are the primary triggering factor that leads to facial pain of muscle origin.

John first came for treatment in 1989 with the main complaint of intense pain in an upper right molar that increased with chewing. He consistently avoided the right side of his mouth while chewing, and had convinced himself that he needed either a new filling or a root canal procedure. An examination found no problems with his teeth, and x-rays revealed nothing of concern. John's facial muscles were extremely tender, however. When he was asked to bring his teeth together, his jaw muscles bulged. When asked whether his teeth were in contact during the day he quickly responded, saying, "All the time, shouldn't they?"

A bit of probing revealed that John was new to New York City and trying to work his way up in the commercial video business. He was employed by a particularly unpleasant man who demanded a 60-hour week for a meager salary. Making ends meet was no easy task, and with few hours to exercise, relax, or sleep, John felt his world was out of control. As a result, he was making a "fist in his face." He did this not only during the hours of work, which often extended to Saturday and Sunday, but he even woke up with his "teeth plastered together." John was admittedly upset about his plight, and it was not surprising that his fatigued, sore, and overworked muscles were sending out signals of referred pain to his teeth.

Knowing that John had no choice but to keep his job despite the poor pay and extensive hours, what direction of care could possibly work if John remained angry? Treatment initially focused on teaching him how to keep his teeth apart during the day, so that if his muscles were assaulted less they would be less fatigued and, therefore, less capable of referring pain to his teeth. In addition, by teaching John a number of simple jaw exercises, he would be able to diminish the tension in his jaw muscles. At night, an oral appliance, such as a nightguard, was prescribed to diminish the impact of his clenching and allow John to get up in the morning with less compromised muscles.

Despite his anger, the physical challenges to his muscles were reduced as a result of these interventions and, over time, his symptoms were markedly reduced. Though John was still not in control, the realization that his symptoms were being driven by emotions, coupled with a number of supportive interventions, allowed him to no longer need active care.

John eventually bought his own video business and became extremely successful. For over 20 years he was without symptoms, despite no longer wearing his oral appliance and, admittedly, falling back into a pattern of clenching his teeth as a response to managing his growing business and home responsibilities. His jaw muscles clearly bulged as his teeth touched, but he was without symptoms and his muscles were not tender when examined.

At this point, John's story confirmed our suspicion that the mere act of bringing the teeth together forcefully and frequently is often insufficient to generate muscle compromise to the point where pain symptoms emerge. Millions of people live "tooth-to-tooth" during the day and/or clench during the night with no consequences. This resiliency is a testament to the adaptive and recuperative capacities that remain intact and efficient, as long as the brain is not excessively challenged by life's emotions.

John recently came back for treatment, however, complaining of pain in an upper right molar. His pain increased with chewing, and he was back to avoiding the right side of his mouth. Examination of his teeth was unremarkable, but his jaw muscles, which had not been tender for 20 years, were extremely painful when examined. What had happened to John?

John's mother suffered a debilitating stroke and she had to relocate to a nursing home. Concern and attention to his mother's condition, along with work concerns prompted by the economic recession, were likely significant reasons for his brain to become overloaded. His brain, in other words, probably lost its ability to control the neural and circulatory processes that ultimately determine muscle comfort. John summed it up best when he said, "I know that I don't have a tooth problem or disease. I have symptoms that are the result of life getting the better of my emotions."

As discussed in Chapter 5, a brain under siege sets the muscles up for failure, allowing habits or tendencies (e.g., clenching, nail biting), structural relations (e.g., bite relationships, postures), and repetitive work positions—which are tolerated by millions of people on a daily basis—to become significant risk factors for pain. As a result, controlling the emotional issues that set the muscles up for failure is frequently the most critical component of care.

## The Four Levels of Treatment: Understanding, Behavior Change, Physical Treatment, and Medication

Since most facial pain symptoms exist because of muscles that ache as a response to continual life challenges that overload the brain, patients require a blend of treatment strategies to confront the broad dimensions of their problems, which we typically employ in steps or stages.

The first step is to help patients recognize what is fueling their emotions, and then to motivate them to change the way their body responds to these challenges. If your tendency, for example, is to brace your jaw or clench your teeth during the day, then learning to keep your jaw relaxed and teeth apart will help decrease the likelihood that you will suffer from the consequences of fatigued and overworked muscles. Though this strategy seems overly simplistic, it works, but is not as easy to implement as it seems. These are learned postures, and changing them takes time and effort.

For patients who come to us soon after their symptoms start, breaking a longstanding habit may be all that is needed for recovery to occur. For those patients who come for treatment with longstanding symptoms that are due to chronic muscle guarding, active trigger points, and/or sensitization, therapies that work directly with the muscles probably will be required.

Treatment, therefore, can be provided on a number of levels, all of which require the active participation of the patient:

Level 1: Recognizing and accepting that the emotions and challenges of life are most likely the reason why your face hurts.

Level 2: Making life changes that are realistic and obtainable.

Level 3: Changing the way your body is responding to a brain under siege (self-regulation techniques).

Level 4: Participating in treatments that are designed to address the physical changes that have already developed in the muscles.

Unlike a broken leg that will predictably take 8 weeks to fully mend, the time frame for muscles to recover is not well defined. The criteria for success are often subjective. When patients say they feel better, both formal treatment efforts and scheduled visits are reduced. At times, patients cancel a visit, simply stating that they are feeling better and not in need of additional care. Once discharged from treatment, the vast majority of patients are never seen again. Though many may suffer setbacks down the road, it is likely that the skills they learned are sufficient to prevent acute experiences of pain.

## Muscle Treatments

Although understanding the influence of a besieged brain on your pain symptoms is critical to getting better, when muscle tissue becomes sensitized, treatment often must also include working directly with the muscles. In situations where there are no easy answers to the challenges patients face, our goal is to buy time for them so we can limit the progression of physical problems in the muscles. This is when we introduce treatments such as self-regulation techniques, muscle exercises and postural programs, muscle injections, physical therapy, medications, and oral appliances, to complement the conversations and mind-body insights we share with our patients.

## Physical Self-Regulation Techniques

The goal of physical self-regulation (PSR) is to get patients to monitor and control the tension they hold in their jaw, other facial areas, neck, and shoulder muscles. Self-regulatory control is achieved when you have the capacity to override your thoughts, feelings, urges, or behaviors in order to reduce pain and improve function. Some of these skills can be taught by facial pain doctors in the office, or with formal training by psychologists, physical therapists, biofeedback therapists, or other health professionals. Learning these skills is not always easy, and patients commonly put up barriers because of their beliefs and expectations. The end result of physical self-regulation is to produce physiologic changes that reduce pain, fatigue and muscle misuse.

If you want to embrace this effective technique, however, you must learn how to do the following:

- Step 1: Relax your facial, oral, and jaw musculature
- Step 2: Gentle Head Movements
- Step 3: Ease upper back tightness
- Step 4: Take brief relaxation breaks
- Step 5: Learn and implement diaphragmatic breathing patterns
- Step 6: Begin sleep in a relaxed position

Specifically, the steps listed below indicate how to implement physical self-regulation techniques. This routine represents (with slight modifications) the Physical Self Regulation Program developed by P. M. Bertrand and C. R. Carlson (2001).

STEP 1: Relax facial, oral, and jaw muscles
a. Sit straight and relaxed, with knees approximately shoulder width apart and with stomach muscles relaxed.
b. Arms should rest on thighs comfortably with hands open and fingers slightly curled.
c. Head is straight with relaxed neck muscles.
d. Shoulders are relaxed and evenly dropped.
Now relax your lips . . . relax your tongue . . . and keep teeth slightly apart. Remember: lips together, teeth apart. The teeth on a daily basis should only touch during eating. You can achieve this by licking your lips,

93

swallowing, then repeating words beginning with the letter (or sound) "n" or "m" (for example, Nancy, Emma). "If you don't know where to place the tongue just let it rest quietly in your mouth with no pressure on the tip.

STEP 2: Gentle head movements

a. Close your eyes. If this feels uncomfortable leave your eyes open.

b. While practicing lips relaxed, tongue relaxed, teeth slightly apart, exhale through the mouth while slowly flexing head downward (about 4 seconds). Avoid any movement that causes discomfort, tightness or pain.

c. Pause with head comfortably flexed for about 2-3 seconds.

d. Inhale through the nose as you slowly return the head to a non-flexed neutral position (about 4 seconds).

e. Pause 1 second before exhaling and flexing the head downward again.

f. Perform steps (a-e) 6 times in about 1 minute; this should be done 6 times/day every 2.5-3 hours.

These gentle symmetrical head motions help with the even distribution of blood flow.

STEP 3: Gentle arm movements (eases back and shoulder tension)

a. Slowly move the arms forward across the thighs for approximately 5 seconds, and then back to the starting position (5 seconds). The hands should always rest on the thighs.

b. Repeat this arm motion slowly 6 times in about 1 minute and perform this 6 times/day every 2.5-3 hours.

STEP 4: Take brief relaxation breaks

The nature of your work and home situation will largely determine when and how often you are able to take a relaxation break. If you work at a desk, for example, you may want to get up every hour or so to stretch or take a walk, or if you have a sales job that requires you to stand for long periods of time, you may want to sit down every hour or so. Using a signaling device, such as a digital timer, which you can manually set to ring or beep every half hour or hour, can be an invaluable tool to remind you it is time for a relaxation break.

STEP 5: Do diaphragmatic breathing

a. Close your eyes (unless this makes you dizzy) and keep your eyelids and forehead relaxed and smooth.

b. Relax your mouth with lips and teeth apart.

c. Keep your shoulders sloped and even.

d. Bend your elbows.

e. Place your hands on your thighs in a curled position.

f. Keep your knees apart.

g. Proceed as follows: As you bring air into the nose, breathe slowly and regularly with your diaphragm. As you inhale oxygen through the nose, the diaphragm gently raises the stomach. When you exhale carbon dioxide, the stomach will fall as the diaphragm relaxes.

Before inhaling again, try to *pause* comfortably for several seconds. The pause is *not* holding your breath. The pause is time to be still and relax. If at any time you begin to feel lightheaded or dizzy, your air exchange is too high. Return to your normal breathing pattern, or try to pause longer between breaths and do not breathe as deeply.

Diaphragmatic breathing, if done properly, is important because it can reduce the release of stress hormones, promotes muscle relaxation, encourages sleep, and enhances the distribution of oxygen and glucose throughout the body. The optimum delivery of oxygen and glucose depends on effective diaphragmatic breathing.

Pain patients often forget to breathe diaphragmatically. Instead, they tend to breathe rapidly, using upper chest, neck and shoulder muscles primarily. Under such conditions, patients exhale carbon dioxide too quickly and achieve a carbon dioxide deficit (hypocapnia). Hypocapnia should be avoided as it increases stress hormone levels, decreases the availability of oxygen to tissues, tightens muscles, and, in extreme cases, alters blood chemistry. Unless you are participating in strenuous exercise, breathe using your diaphragm.

STEP 6: Begin sleep in a relaxed position to help control nighttime activity such as clenching

a. Lay on your back and put one pillow under your knees and another under your head for support. Practice slow diaphragmatic breathing.

b. Then, say aloud 6-7 times, "teeth apart, lips relaxed, tongue relaxed, sleep relaxed," while picturing yourself sleeping in a relaxed position.

c. Start off sleeping on your back. Don't worry if you move.

## Exercises and Manual Therapy

When you have muscle problems, a regimen of home exercises or more formal hands-on care with a physical therapist, osteopath, massage therapist, or chiropractor may be appropriate. While home exercises are the first line of therapy, referral to an independent practitioner is common. These types of hands-on therapies are designed to restore health to compromised muscles. Without insight into what is driving your muscle dysfunction, however, these efforts will either fail or have short-term benefit. Any practitioner you go to should be well-versed in mind-body interactions and advise you that their manual techniques alone will be unlikely to cure your symptoms. If their efforts can help break your cycle of pain, and facilitate the restoration of normal muscle physiology, then you will suffer less and be able to spend more energy on addressing the true sources of your problems.

Our preference over the years has been to refer patients to practitioners who not only possess exceptional hands-on manual skills that effectively and predictably lead to muscle recovery, but who set aside ample time to listen to patients and address the mind–body connections that are so critical to the recovery process. Their emotional support is an essential component to the care they provide. If, in fact, the fascial system (see pages 40-41)—which is responsible for muscle structure and protection—is, as physical therapist John F. Barnes believes, "The reservoir of our emotions," then treatment goals become very clear. Manual therapy must engage the fascia in an effort to restore muscle health, and conversation must be ongoing so that patients fully appreciate the effort, insight and participation that is required of them (e.g., the 60/40 rule) on a daily basis. These manual therapies are often critical in jump-starting muscle recovery, and vary in duration based on the multiple factors that may have initiated and or perpetuated the muscle compromises.

## Jaw and Neck Exercises

The following exercises are often helpful to patients with facial pain, but they do not represent the full scope of options available. Remember to breathe normally as you do the exercises. You should not experience any pain while doing them.

Jaw Exercise 1
Goal: Release tension in jaw-closing muscles
Place your thumb directly under your chin. Place your tongue on the roof of your mouth, halfway back. Attempt to open your mouth against gentle thumb resistance, as your tongue is kept in contact with the roof of your mouth. Resist for 3-4 seconds without letting your jaw reach the maximum open position. Repeat 6 times.

Jaw Exercise 2
Goal: Stretch jaw-closing muscles
While sitting down, place your left elbow on a table and lean your forehead into the palm of your hand. With the index and middle fingers of your right hand, pull down on the lower front teeth to open the jaw until you feel a stretch in your facial muscles. Hold for 3-4 seconds, release, and repeat 10 times.

Jaw Exercise 3
Goal: Help coordination of muscles that move jaw from side to side
Take a tongue blade (given to you by your doctor) and gently rest it between your upper and lower teeth. Swing your jaw to the right, gliding on the tongue blade, and feel the resistance. Hold it for 3-4 seconds. Repeat on the opposite side. Do 10 repetitions of both.

Jaw Exercise 4
Goal: Limit forward movement of jaw on mouth opening
Place your tongue on the roof of your mouth, halfway back. Open your mouth in front of a mirror. Try to open it in a straight line. Hold it in a limited open position for 5 seconds. Release. Repeat 5-10 times.

Neck Exercise 1

Goal: Gentle stretch of upper neck muscles

Sit in a chair with your feet on the ground. Anchor your right hand under the chair. Turn your head to the left and place your left hand on the back of your head. Pull your head down towards your left shoulder with gentle force. Turn your nose into your armpit for increased stretch of the trapezius muscle. Hold 3-4 seconds. Relax. Reverse the exercise and repeat on the other side. Repeat 10 times on each side.

Neck Exercise 2

Goal: Gentle stretch of upper neck muscles

Sit in a chair with your feet on the ground. Anchor your right hand under the chair. Turn your head to the left and place your left hand across your left temple. Gently pull backwards stretching your lateral neck muscle (sternocleidomastoid). Hold 3-4 seconds. Repeat 10 times. Reverse directions to stretch the opposite side.

Neck Exercise 3

Goal: Gentle stretch of upper neck muscles

Clasp your hands over your head, and pull your head down gently, chin to chest. Hold 5 seconds. Release. Repeat 10 times.

Remember to breathe throughout all of these exercises. You should not feel any pain as you move through the routine.

## Posture

Though we do not feel that poor posture as an independent factor is responsible for the onset of persistent facial pain problems (just like tooth grinding and clenching often occur without pain symptoms developing), it must be considered a risk factor when coupled with a brain "under siege." For this reason, home programs to address postural strains can provide relief when routinely practiced. The specifics of these programs are best determined subsequent to evaluation by a trained manual therapist.

## Medications

When we manage patients in pain, the use of medications varies for each individual. Using medications for acute muscle pain or flare-ups of chronic muscle conditions is common. Medication is rarely the primary focus of treatment, but often can help start the process towards recovery or instill optimism in difficult situations. Medications can be used to reduce pain, muscle contracture, and inflammation; assist the sleep process; and bolster the body's own pain-relieving systems. They can be administered orally, topically, or via injection. With our approach to treatment, when patients with muscle pain are prescribed medications, they are constantly reminded to look inward for the answers and not to rely on a few pills for relief. The variety, duration, and frequency of medications prescribed for patients vary considerably, as follows:

### Pain Medications

Mild to moderate pain can be treated with oral medications such as acetaminophen (e.g., Tylenol). All medication for pain should be taken on a regular schedule, rather than as needed, in order to maximize its potential to control pain symptoms. Topical creams and patches also can be helpful for pain control. The use of anti-inflammatory medication, such as aspirin, ibuprofen (e.g., Advil) or naproxen (e.g., Aleve) for pain is also common, but must be used with caution over an extended period of time (see the discussion immediately below). Narcotic medications are not usually used to manage pain of muscle origin.

Most of the time, pain medication is not the focal point of treatment. Essentially, it buys some time as other therapies are integrated into the overall treatment plan. These medications can be taken during the day or just prior to bedtime, depending on the symptoms. At times, a combination of anti-inflammatory medication and acetaminophen-based products are taken together to assist in pain reduction.

### Anti-Inflammatory Medications

Anti-inflammatory medications can be used to manage any type of mild to moderate pain, but they are most helpful for pain that is due to inflammation. Muscles certainly can be compromised by persistent inflammation, and medications can control the symptoms. Finding out what is causing

99

the inflammation is critical before treatment to stop the inflammation begins.

As with pain medications, anti-inflammatory medications must be used on a schedule in order to be effective. Whether they are used once, twice, or four times a day depends on both the cause of the inflammation and the likelihood the patient will follow the treatment recommendations. Since inflammation is often the engine that drives further tissue injury or nerve excitation, these medications at times need to be taken for one to several months in order to be effective. All anti-inflammatory medications can cause gastrointestinal upset, promote excessive bleeding, and compromise kidney function over time. Caution is therefore required with long-term use.

## Muscle Relaxants

Muscle relaxants can work either directly on muscle tissue or they can exert their action in the brain to reduce muscle contracture. Muscle relaxants have limited usefulness during the daytime hours, but can be taken prior to bedtime to reduce the intensity of parafunctional activities, such as clenching and tooth grinding. On a short-term basis, these medications seem to be helpful in promoting more restful sleep. Patients who use them often feel as if their neck and jaw muscles are less tight when they wake up. After using muscle relaxants for a long period of time, however, they can lose their effectiveness. When this happens, it is common for medications to be switched. Patients who take these medications may feel a bit groggy and sluggish in the morning. If this lingers more than an hour or so, changes in the dosage or type of medication should be made. During the day, these medications seem to be too sedative for consistent use.

## Anti-Anxiety Drugs as Muscle Relaxants

This class of medications has been used for years, primarily at bedtime to decrease the intensity of parafunctional activity (clenching/grinding) at night. While they are often helpful initially, their effectiveness decreases with time. This makes it necessary to increase the dosage. Dependence on these medications can occur over time, but sometimes the benefits outweigh the risks.

During the day, these medications are most useful for decreasing generalized anxiety and the accompanying muscle bracing and contracture that follow. Patients often find that these medications diminish the neck and jaw muscle contraction that typically follows a stressful work or home encounter or an unpleasant or worrisome thought. These medications are most likely to be profoundly helpful when a behavioral psychologist or psycho-pharmacologist is part of an overall plan of treatment. Because a brain under siege can drive muscle problems, we often combine medications and cognitive strategies designed to address anxiety and the issues that accompany it.

## Medications to Diminish Nerve Sensitization

When muscles have been dysfunctional for long periods of time, it is common for the nerves that run through the muscle fibers to become irritated. As a result, the threshold for these nerves to fire is markedly reduced. As this continues, the muscle pain cycle is reinforced. To confront this vicious cycle, a number of medications are used to reduce nerve discharge. These medications, like many of the others discussed here, are typically used in conjunction with other therapies.

For patients who have suffered for a long period of time, we sometimes consider medications that can bolster the body's own pain-blunting systems. These medications have been used for years to manage a variety of pain problems that have multiple origins. They have been shown to increase naturally-occurring endorphins and reduce nerve discharge, and are typically well tolerated if started in small doses and increased over time as symptoms dictate. In many cases, we use pharmacies to customize the dosage of these medications so that benefit can be achieved without the typical side effects that might discourage use.

## Topical and Transdermal Medications

Whether the goal is to reduce inflammation, diminish the perception of pain, or control the firing of nerve endings, there are a number of topical and transdermal medications that are often helpful adjuncts in the treatment of patients' problems. Topical medications, applied as a cream or salve, mostly affect only the areas on which they are applied. If they are used frequently, however, they can get into the blood circulation and lead to side effects. Transdermal medications, most often used in the form of a "patch," are released slowly over time, allowing greater therapeutic benefit and more potential side effects. Patches can be worn under garments in the neck and shoulder region during the day, as well as at night while you sleep.

Available over-the-counter or obtained through prescriptions, topical and transdermal medications typically contain local anesthetic, anti-inflammatory agents, and medications that dampen nerve discharge. Unless skin reactions develop they can be used over long periods of time, either alone (if oral medications cannot be tolerated) or to complement oral medications or injections.

## Medications for Sleep

Anything that can improve the quality and quantity of a patient's sleep is a priority, since adequate sleep is critical for muscle tissue to heal. Because sleep problems can be complex, additional medical consultation is sometimes necessary to insure that a patient receives a comprehensive plan of action. Medications are certainly one of many options available, and may be essential to obtain the sleep that is necessary for healing to occur.

## Natural Supplements and Homeopathic Remedies

For patients who are uncomfortable taking prescription medication, there are a number of natural supplements and homeopathic remedies that appear to produce positive outcomes. Though the results can be unpredictable, a growing body of scientific research supports the use of these alternative options to treat inflammation, muscle tension, and pain.

## Muscle Injections

Some patients benefit from muscle trigger-point injections, a treatment technique that can be administered with a dry needle or a local anesthetic solution. These injections are designed to release muscle tension from compromised muscles. They are effective because of the mechanical prodding of the muscle fibers, not the anesthetic, if one is used. The anesthetic makes the procedure less uncomfortable and may reduce the soreness in the muscle over the following few days. Steroids like cortisone are not routinely used during trigger-point therapy, but if there is a tendonitis condition, a steroid may be injected.

As we discussed in Chapter 3, these injection techniques also have been shown to reduce the ability of muscles to refer pain. The case of Ken is a good example of the efficacy of muscle injections for facial pain.

When 57-year-old Ken came to the office, he described a continuous ache located specifically in the gum tissues near the upper right eye tooth. Despite numerous dental interventions, which included bite adjustments, the replacement of a crown, "exploratory" gum surgery, and medications for nerve pain, Ken's symptoms continued. Upon hearing his history, further diagnosis and evaluation revealed that his right temporalis muscle was in a state of contracture—tense and sore. After a series of injections into the body of the muscle, Ken's symptoms eased and then disappeared. His persistent symptoms and demand for care resulted in unsuccessful treatment from others, because their treatment was directed to the location of the pain, not the source.

Muscle injections can be administered in the facial muscles and neck muscles, and are complemented by home techniques to stretch the treated muscles. At times, muscle tendons are the culprits when pain symptoms have lingered for a long period of time. In some instances, the use of steroid injections into the tendons is necessary to prompt a process of recovery. Tendon injections in the facial and jaw muscles are no different than those given in other body parts, and must be supported by other forms of therapy.

## Botox

This popular "muscle paralyzer" is used to buy time for patients under certain circumstances. Unquestionably, we are sometimes faced with difficult muscle pain problems that have been present for long periods and have origins for which there are no easy or immediate answers. Many of the patients with these problems have practiced self-regulation techniques and tried a variety of treatments, including medications, exercises, physical therapy, oral appliances, and counseling, but continue to suffer. In these cases, Botox injections may be chosen as an alternative form of therapy.

Since Botox has the capacity to partially incapacitate the ability of a muscle to contract, it provides an ideal option for patients who have not responded to more common forms of therapy. These injections can be administered in jaw and other facial muscles and neck muscles. If effective, they will reduce muscle tension and symptoms for 2-4 months. During this time, the muscles and their tendons are given an opportunity to heal, as reduced tension allows increased blood flow, bringing the nutrients and oxygen necessary for cellular repair. Occasionally, repeat injections are necessary. Breaking the cycle of pain and dysfunction is the ultimate goal of care and, for some, Botox is an appropriate option.

## Oral Appliances

For patients who clench and/or grind their teeth while sleeping, oral appliances (nightguards) are utilized. A modified version of this device may be used during the day to create awareness of a destructive behavior. During sleep they are designed to diminish the impact of grinding or clenching. Though research has not fully identified why these appliances work, patients often experience significant relief from wearing them. They are often indispensible in helping to manage pain, muscle tightness, and unstable jaw joints for patients who have a true TMJ condition.

These appliances are best obtained from dentists, who will custom fit the device for a specific problem. Over-the-counter devices, for the most part, are either inadequate for reducing symptoms or they aggravate the muscle or joint problem. For patients who have facial muscle pain but no evidence of overbuilt muscles or worn tooth surfaces, there is little justification for using these devices. Where there is justification for making an oral appliance, patients may use them either short-term or for an extended, undefined period of time. In the vast majority of cases, these appliances are not made with the intent of moving teeth, changing the bite, or altering a patient's jaw position.

## Biofeedback Training

Biofeedback is a means for gaining control of your body processes to increase relaxation, relieve pain, and develop healthier, more comfortable life patterns. With biofeedback, you obtain information about yourself by means of external instruments. Using a thermometer to take your temperature, for example, is a common type of biofeedback. Clinical biofeedback follows the same principle. Specialized instruments are used to monitor various physiological processes as they occur. Moving graphs on a computer screen and audio tones that go up and down "reflect" changes as they occur in the body system being measured.

The main function of biofeedback training is to familiarize you with the activity in your various body systems, so you may learn to control the activity to relieve stress and improve health. Trying to change physiological activity without biofeedback is like playing darts while blindfolded—you can't see whether you are hitting the mark or not. Biofeedback lets you know precisely when you are changing your physiological functions or processes in the desired direction.

Biofeedback is not a treatment. Rather, it is an educational process for learning specialized mind-body skills. Learning to recognize physiological responses and alter them is not unlike learning how to play the piano or tennis—it requires practice. Through practice, you become familiar with your own unique psychophysiological patterns and responses to stress, and learn to control them rather than having them control you (Schwartz & Andrasik, 2003)

## Cognitive-Behavioral Therapy

Cognitive-behavioral therapy (CBT) is a form of psychotherapy that emphasizes the important role that thinking has on how you feel and what you do (Craske, 2009). CBT is based on the idea that your feelings and behaviors are caused by your thoughts, not by external factors, like people, situations, and events. The benefit of this approach is that you can change the way you think in order to feel better, even if the situation does not change.

As discussed throughout this book, many of our patients over the years have needed help to develop insight into how their lives impact their muscles. "Talk therapy" can be critical in helping patients turn that corner when other forms of treatment have fallen short. In situations where medication is needed to address anxiety, depression, or other persistent concerns, we refer patients to a psychiatrist or psycho-pharmacologist (see the previous section on anti-anxiety medications). As we have said, the vast majority of our patients do not require formal counseling or psychotherapy. Providing our patients with insight into the mind-body connection and giving them the tools to change destructive tendencies and rehabilitate their muscles is most often what is required.

## Summary

Many options exist to treat facial pain. In this chapter, we have discussed the importance of first listening to patients, validating their symptoms, and encouraging their participation in the treatment process (the 60/40 rule). After diagnosing each patient, we use one or more of four levels of treatment to relieve the pain and/or suffering they are experiencing, including understanding, behavior change, physical treatment, and medication.

Finding the best treatment for a given patient requires obtaining a personal and medical history, a physical examination, and insight into the patient's world. In this process, we find it helpful to characterize each patient as being in one of three possible patient profile groups, including those with pain from everyday life challenges, those with pain from a brain under siege, or those with pain who have no muscle dysfunction.

The success we have had with the majority of our patients over the years is attributable to the treatment strategies that we have implemented. A combination of knowledge, patient participation, and carefully selected treatments continues to be a winning formula.

Throughout the course of every year, most facial pain patients exhibit signs and symptoms that seem to represent a typical case of muscular dysfunction. At times, however, some patients do not get better, and both the character of their complaints and their physical profile changes. In these instances, alternative diagnoses need to be considered and other medical practitioners should be consulted. Chapter 7 addresses these situations—when things are not what they seem to be.

## Chapter 7

# WHEN THINGS ARE NOT WHAT THEY SEEM TO BE

*Your face, my thane, is as a book where men may read strange matters.* — Shakespeare, *Macbeth*

Among the patients we have treated over the years, some have reported familiar symptoms such as "My face hurts," "I can't open my mouth widely," and "I have an intense headache." With careful listening, however, their symptom description, history, and clinical presentation suggested that something was different. Though symptoms were being expressed through the muscles it was unlikely that emotions and learned behaviors were the culprits. In such instances, further investigation is required, which often reveals an underlying medical cause. At other times, early failure of routine treatment strategies directed towards the muscles encourages reassessment and the consideration of alternative diagnoses in the search for answers. In this concluding chapter, we discuss several of these enigmatic, complex, and sometimes inexplicable cases.

## Intense Tooth Pain without Tooth Pathology

Our encounters with patients over the last 25 years have revealed one specific subset of patients that reflects a difficult diagnostic dilemma. They describe constant toothache pain in one or more teeth but have no jaw or other facial pain complaints. Typically, they say that their tooth pain came on spontaneously and increased slowly in intensity over time. Unlike typical tooth pain symptoms, their pain does not increase with hot or cold food or liquids and often stays the same when chewing. Despite the severity of their constant pain, their dental x-rays are unremarkable and clinical examinations do not reveal any clear tooth compromise. Due to the severity of the pain, the patient often convinces his or her dentist to treat a specific tooth or teeth, which results in both more pain and a broadening of the painful area.

As this scenario unfolds, it becomes clear that the patient does not have true tooth pathology. In addition, the constant nature and description of the pain (gnawing, burning) makes it unlikely that the patient is suffering from either classic trigeminal neuralgia (see later in this chapter) or pain of muscle origin. In addition, the symptoms are clearly not the result of emotional suffering.

These patients are likely in trouble as a result of nerve excitation that occurs and persists for no apparent reason. For some of these patients, normal oral stimuli leads to the perception of pain, whether it is the touching of the teeth with the lips, the biting down on food, or the movement of the tongue against the teeth or gum tissue. For others, constant pain is reported with no additional pain prompted by chewing or oral stimulation. In essence it seems that, in these scenarios, nerve endings fire more readily for reasons that cannot often be identified. As a result, these patients often complain of tooth pain when there is little evidence to support a diagnosis of tooth pathology.

As a result of the patient's description of the pain intensity, his or her dentist is apt to interpret a shadow on an x-ray as significant and indicative of decay, when that same shadow would have been overlooked in a patient without pain symptoms who came in for a routine cleaning. In addition, deep fillings are often blamed for symptoms when those same fillings would likely be left alone in another patient without pain symptoms. Here is a striking case history that provides a classic example of this type of problem.

Christine was 43 years old when she came in for treatment. Her primary symptom was persistent pain in two upper right back teeth, which she had been experiencing for approximately 10 months. Her pain had come on spontaneously and increased with chewing. Although there was no clear-cut evidence of tooth compromise, before Christine came to us she had a root canal procedure that not only increased tooth pain intensity, but caused the pain to spread to a neighboring tooth. In addition, Christine's gums started to burn. Convinced that the pain must be due to the neighboring tooth that was now hurting, Christine insisted that "something must be done to ease her pain." As a result of her cries for help and insistence that her pain must be coming from her teeth, her dentist provided additional treatment. The second molar was treated with root canal therapy and the molar that had been treated with root canal initially was extracted, easing Christine's pain for 1 week before it re-emerged.

By this time, Christine was, in her own words, "mentally worn down." Despite all the unsuccessful dental treatment, she was convinced that her problems were still in her teeth. She had also consulted with her primary care physician, two neurologists, an otolaryngologist, and several dental specialists. She was tired of hearing "there is nothing wrong with you," as she continued to suffer. She also recognized that it had been her cry for help, and not the examination findings of the dentists, that led to treatment. She took responsibility for the direction that care had taken because "I just wanted to feel better." Christine's problem, however, was most likely due to the loss of regulation in the discharge or interpretation of oral nerve activity, and not related to her teeth at all.

Christine's story represents a situation where things were not what they seemed to be. It is just one example of a case that taught us that dental intervention should be avoided in the absence of clear-cut examination and x-ray findings. At the present time, though we continue to struggle with assigning an absolute diagnosis to these problems, it is our sense that these tooth-site pain symptoms are likely due to a lowered firing threshold of nerve endings in the mouth/teeth (leading to excessive nerve firing), and/or the interpretation of normal nerve signals sent to the brain as noxious.

As a result, the primary treatment options include the use of a variety of oral and topical medications to challenge the overall pain experience by diminishing nerve discharge and, at the same time, diminishing the brain's perception of incoming nerve signals. With time, treatments proved successful in making Christine feel better, but not totally free from pain symptoms. Most importantly, Christine understood that her tooth pains were not related to the teeth, and she no longer demanded treatment when her symptoms occasionally flared. From her perspective, she hoped that dentists and physicians eventually would become more aware of problems like hers and acknowledge that tooth pain can be present even in the absence of a recognizable tooth problem. From our perspective, such awareness among our medical and dental colleagues would go a long way towards reducing unfavorable and sometimes pain-exacerbating outcomes that often follow misdirected treatment.

## Facial Pain Caused by Underlying Medical Problems

Pain can emerge in the mouth, jaw, and other facial areas as a result of medical problems associated with the salivary glands, heart, inflammatory conditions—involving blood vessels, neuralgias, thyroid disease, intracranial tumors (located in the head)—and a host of other conditions.

Clues are often subtle that suggest the cause of facial pain is a problem unrelated to muscles or teeth, but they usually reveal themselves over the course of time. Several factors that may distinguish a common facial pain problem from one associated with a more serious medical issue include the following:

1. Facial pain that is constant, but does not necessarily increase with eating, opening and closing of the mouth, or head movements requiring contraction of the neck muscles

2. Persistent ear pain that never eases and is unresponsive to treatment

3. Exacerbation of facial pain with talking, smiling, or exertional actions, such as sneezing or coughing

4. Facial pain that is described with the words "excruciating," "sickening," or "twitching"

5. Facial pain that is accompanied by visual changes, deficits in hearing, and changes in taste and/or smell

6. Facial pain that is accompanied by a profound and persistent sense of numbness or tingling in the tongue, lower lip, or face

7. Vague facial pain on the left or right side of the jaw and upper neck that does not increase with jaw function but does increase with physical activity or efforts

8. A quick onset of extreme jaw muscle fatigue and a sense of weakness within moments of starting to chew

9. A marked, gradual change in the way the teeth come together without apparent cause

10. Absence of any type of response after 6-8 weeks of treatment directed at the jaw and neck muscles

11. The presence of facial swelling, with or without accompanying pain

Though these factors are not always associated with a problem of medical concern, it is wise for individuals to pursue additional medical consultation if any of them persist for more than 1 or 2 months.

## Facial Neuralgias

Neuralgia is pain in one or more nerves produced by a change in neurological structure or function, rather than by the excitation of pain receptor cells located, for instance, in the gums, skin or teeth. Facial neuralgias are rare, with only about 4 cases for every 100,000 people, whereas the facial pain problems of muscle origin we have focused on occur in about 4 out of 100 people (Lipton, Ship, & Larach-Robinson, 1993). When facial neuralgias do occur, however, patients often have intense moments of facial pain, such as toothache and jaw pain, or jaw muscle spasm that limits mouth opening.

*Trigeminal neuralgia* is a particularly painful facial neuralgia. This disorder of the trigeminal nerve (a cranial nerve) causes short-lived attacks of severe pain in the lips, cheeks, gums, or chin on one side of the face. About 30-40% of patients diagnosed with trigeminal neuralgia experience toothache pain as the most common first symptom.

Trigeminal neuralgia occurs most often in women, typically comes on after the age of 50, and is commonly associated with periods of both debilitating pain and remission. The pain of trigeminal neuralgia is typically not constant, comes on in waves, and lasts only a few seconds before totally disappearing. Patients with trigeminal neuralgia may experience debilitating pain for 20 seconds and then absolute comfort for minutes, hours, or even days. Many patients report the spontaneous emergence of pain ("I was sitting at my desk reading when excruciating and sharp pain radiated through my face into my lip and teeth"), while others report a pain onset provoked by talking, eating, brushing teeth, combing hair, putting on makeup, or even a gust of wind.

Trigeminal neuralgia is characterized as either idiopathic or symp-tomatic. Idiopathic neuralgias may not have an identifiable origin, while those characterized as symptomatic may be due to multiple sclerosis, diseases influencing the structure of nerve tissue, or intracranial pathology, including aggressive, large tumors. Typically, these problems are managed medically or surgically.

The case of Shirley, 60 years old, illustrates a patient with pain due to trigeminal neuralgia. She described the presence of sharp bouts of intense, sporadic facial pain that radiated into her teeth and jaws. The pain could come on with talking or eating, or emerge spontaneously without provocation. Most importantly, Shirley noted that, although the pain and facial muscle spasm could be intense, these symptoms often disappeared totally for hours or days at a time. As quickly as symptoms had emerged or became more intense, they stopped or became less intense. Shirley had prior treatment, including root canal therapy on one tooth, the placement of a mouth guard to address "clenching," and anti-inflammatory medication, but all of these procedures had limited impact on the pattern and intensity of her pain.

The history that Shirley provided and the symptoms she described clearly pointed to a trigeminal neuralgia condition. As a full medical evaluation did not reveal pathology that required surgery, it was decided that the appropriate treatment was medication to halt nerve discharge.

## Facial Pain and the Heart

When people experience a heart attack or other cardiac issue, they typically have vague and inconsistent symptoms of facial pain or discomfort. Aside from chest pain, facial pain is, in fact, the most frequent symptom associated with a heart attack. Specifically, 40% of people who experience heart attacks report facial pain, and women experience facial pain more frequently than men during a heart attack. The facial pain symptoms that occur with a cardiac event typically do not increase significantly with jaw movement but can sometimes increase during physical exertion.

Most patients we have seen with facial pain associated with an impending cardiac event were over the age of 45, and they had no or little prior history of jaw problems or common cardiac risk factors, such as high blood pressure. Such patients do not seem to fit any particular facial pain profile and, therefore, they raise doubts regarding their diagnosis and treatment.

Sixty-three-year-old George was one such case. He spoke of left facial and jaw pain that was variable in its presence and character. Some days were better than others, but for no particular reason. He was able to fully open and close his mouth without limitation and did not report increased pain levels with chewing. He was in the midst of having a number of crown restorations replaced on the left side of his mouth, and had been reassured by his dentist that, as soon as his bite was "perfect," his symptoms would disappear. Further questioning revealed that he had never before experienced similar symptoms, and was puzzled by his dentist's diagnosis of tight jaw muscles when, in fact, he was retired and living without any stressful life circumstances. These factors, plus an unremarkable exam that revealed limited muscle pain, prompted a referral for a full medical exam, which George had not had in almost 3 years. An abnormal EKG led to a more complete cardiac evaluation and the discovery of a 75% blockage in an artery on the left side of his heart. Following angioplasty and the placement of a cardiac stent, George's facial pain symptoms disappeared.

## Temporal Arteritis and Facial Pain

Temporal arteritis involves a problem with the blood vessels that serve the craniofacial region. Early on, this condition looks like a typical facial muscle or temporomandibular problem in many ways. Patients often report headache pains in the temples, tight and painful jaw muscles, restricted jaw motion, and an increase in symptoms during chewing. In addition, these patients often describe aches and pains in the upper neck and shoulder region, and examination in this area reveals exquisite soreness of the muscles. Distinguishing characteristics that help identify this problem include the age of the patient (typically late 50s and beyond), a feeling of malaise or generally not feeling well, and the complaint that the jaw fatigues quickly when chewing. In fact, many of these patients report that they can't even eat a piece of bread, as their jaw feels exhausted and weak. If this diagnosis is missed, there can be permanent partial or complete loss of vision on the symptomatic side.

Helen is a typical example of a patient with temporal arteritis who came for treatment, feeling she had just about run out of options. At 70 year of age, she had been experiencing a number of jaw, tooth, and other facial pain symptoms for several months. Despite interventions with her dentist and family doctor, she continued to experience symptoms of varying intensity. On the day she came for a consultation, her appearance suggested that not only was she in pain, but that she was also suffering and not feeling well in general. For the most part, Helen's complaints did not seem that different from those experienced by people with classic TMJ problems, but she winced when the muscles of her upper neck were gently examined, remarking, "I never knew those muscles hurt so much." When asked how she was doing with eating, she quickly responded, "I have lost my appetite in the last few weeks, as my jaw tires terribly when I start to eat." With this comment, it was clear that Helen did not have a jaw problem, but was suffering with temporal arteritis. The diagnosis was confirmed with a blood test and a follow-up biopsy of her temporal artery, which led to the appropriate medical care.

## Head and Neck Tumors

During the course of every year, a few patients who initially appear to have facial pain of muscle origin invariably have tumors associated with the salivary glands, the pharynx, neck vessels, ear, thyroid gland, and brain. When these lesions are in their early stages of development, the symptoms and physical findings appear to be common and benign. As time passes, however, they change, suggesting that things are not what they appear to be. The following are a few cases that will help outline the symptoms and physical findings that should prompt concern.

### *Parotid Tumors*

The parotid gland is the main salivary gland, and it provides most of the saliva that fills our mouths. Located at the angle of the jaw, it extends upward towards the temporomandibular joint and laterally on the face, submerged under the back end of the masseter muscle. Throughout the parotid gland, there are multiple fibers of the seventh nerve (facial nerve) that are responsible for the normal functioning of the muscles of facial expression. When tumors develop in the parotid gland, most are benign but a small percentage are aggressive in nature. They typically grow slowly and, if deep in their location, do not reveal themselves clinically, even though symptoms may have been present for quite some time.

Many patients with parotid tumors complain of persistent ear pain that does not resolve with medication or treatments to the ears or sinuses. The ear pain characteristically becomes more severe with time and is almost always associated with a diminished ability to open the mouth. These patients almost always talk about a slow onset of diminished jaw opening, and this symptom is sometimes associated with vague toothache pain that eludes diagnosis. Regardless of the age of such patients, with these symptoms and a history that cannot explain why they seem to have a jaw problem (no trauma, no overuse habits, no significant life events, no recent dental work), an evaluation of the parotid is essential.

Thirty-year-old Mary was a patient with the classic symptoms of a parotid tumor. She had intense daily right jaw pain that came on spontaneously and had been present for the better part of 1 year. Her jaw range of motion was severely restricted and all attempts to produce wider opening with medication, stretching, oral appliance therapy, and physical therapy had been unsuccessful. Mary reported daily high levels of ear pain that had gotten worse over time, but past medical evaluations did not reveal any significant findings. An examination revealed exquisite tenderness over the facial muscles from the temple down to the lower jaw. An MRI image of the temporomandibular joints was normal, suggesting that motion restriction had to have its origin in the muscles. Based on the spontaneous onset of symptoms 1 year earlier, unresponsiveness to care, persistent and progressive ear pain, and rigid and restricted jaw motion, Mary was sent for additional head and neck imaging, which revealed a tumor in the deep lobe of the parotid gland. Surgical and medical care led to a positive outcome, and over time all jaw symptoms disappeared.

## Intracranial Tumors

Headaches and pain in the jaw and other facial areas can be experienced as a result of intracranial tumors, or tumors that are within the part of the skull that encloses the brain. The reason for these symptoms is that the tumor exerts pressure on the trigeminal nerve (discussed earlier in this chapter). Pain may be felt above the eyebrow, between the eye and upper lip, and in the lower jaw, either independently or in combination.

These patients often have facial pain upon physical exertion, a complaint we take very seriously, since this symptom is unusual in most patients who come for consultation. Other possible signs of this type of tumor are symptoms involving the trigeminal nerve (pain and restricted jaw motion) and the facial nerve (altered facial expressions) that occur at the same time. When this is evident, the likelihood of an intracranial mass is increased.

Sometimes pain is not an issue, but the key symptom is alteration in hearing perception. Common muscle and joint problems do not produce hearing deficits or profoundly clogged ears, as a general rule. Though tinnitus (ringing in the ears) and dizziness may be associated with a common facial muscle or TMD problem, these symptoms always warrant medical scrutiny. The same is true for visual, taste, and/or speaking deficits or changes.

Sixty-year-old Mindy was a patient who returned for treatment with new symptoms 3 years after having been successfully treated for a muscle problem in her face and upper neck.

She reported that over the last month or so her facial pain and muscle tightness had re-emerged on the right side of her face but minimally on the left, which varied from her past experience. She felt at times that her facial muscles would twitch on the right, leading to additional muscle tension. Her physical examination did not suggest any-thing of additional concern, but questioning revealed that over the last 2 months Mindy had experienced a noticeable level of hearing deficit on the right side. Concerned with this symptom and the twitching in her face, she was referred to an ear, nose, and throat specialist. A hearing test revealed a 40% hearing loss in her right ear. A full evaluation along with imaging uncovered an acoustic neuroma (a benign tumor), which if left unattended could have resulted in permanent hearing loss and more significant medical problems.

## Summary

Most people with facial pain find themselves in trouble as a result of benign muscular factors that are most often fueled by emotions and challenging life circumstances and experiences. At times, however, significant medical problems in their early stages of development can cause facial pain symptoms, including facial neuralgias, heart conditions, temporal arteritis, and head and neck tumors. This chapter has attempted to shed some light on the subtle and more obvious signs that help uncover underlying medical issues long before they develop into serious, more difficult-to-manage problems.

# EPILOGUE

As we simultaneously ponder what the future may bring for those suffering with persistent facial pain problems and appreciate that the world of medical science will continue to bring innovation and technology to the examining room, the question of whether this will this lead to more accurate diagnosis and better care remains unclear. In a relatively recent television advertisement that features generations of doctors hovering over an ill child and saying "Let's take a look," we are led to believe that with the advent of new medical technology answers for our patients' complaints and concerns will be more readily uncovered. Though this may have great application in the presence of disease and overt tissue pathology, for the facial pain patient whose presentation often reveals high levels of suffering and few clinical findings one wonders whether the words "Let's listen" continue to make the most sense. If so, then it is incumbent on our professional education system to not only make our healthcare providers better listeners but also to prepare them to ask the right questions.

In this light, medical and dental practitioners—who will remain the first line in evaluating this population of pain patients—must be given a pain education that both encompasses the broad concepts of pain reception, transmission, perception and response *and* focuses on the unique anatomic and neurologic features of the face. For medical schools this will be a daunting task, since currently only limited curriculum time is devoted to the understanding of pain, and even less to the oral cavity, temporomandibular joints and jaw muscles. Dental schools face similar challenges, as current efforts of teaching the concepts of pain have not been universally established, and long-held biases about the origin of facial pain problems remain deeply entrenched. Moving beyond these limit-ations is a challenge that must be realized. Fortunately current efforts in dentistry to establish a specialty in orofacial pain is gaining momentum, which signifies that this serious problem is finally receiving the attention it requires.

# EPILOGUE

It is our final hope that through the collaborative efforts of healthcare practitioners around the world, care for these patients will continue to improve in the years to come. In this regard the "mind–body connection" must continually be recognized, and interested practitioners must be prepared to use their eyes, ears, brain and heart if they hope to help patients suffering with facial pain. Ultimately, however, when trying to determine who will be responsible for these patients, a quote from a psychiatry colleague remains germane. When asked who was the best doctor to treat the facial pain patient, he quickly replied, "an empathetic one." Based on who comes through our doors on a daily basis, we couldn't agree more.

# REFERENCES

Benoliel, Rafael & Sharav,Yair. (2008). Masticatory myofascial pain and tension type and chronic daily headache. In Sharav, Y. & Benoliel, R. (eds.). *Orofacial Pain & Headache* (pp. 109-148). London: Mosby.

Bonica, John. (1953). *The management of pain.* Phila., PA: Lippincott, Williams & Wilkins.

Bertrand, P. M. & Carlson, C. R. (2001). *Physical Self Regulation.* A handout. Orofacial Pain Center, NPDS, Bethesda, MD and Orofacial Pain Center, UK, Lexington, KY.

Cahill, Cheryl & Akil, Huda (2006). Plasma beta-endorphin-like immunoreactivity, self reported pain perception and anxiety levels in women during pregnancy and labor. *Life Sciences, 31*(16-17), 1871-1873.

Carlson, C. R., Bertrand, P. M., Ehrlich, A. D., Maxwell, A. W. & Burton, R. G. (2001). Physical self-regulation training for the management of temporomandibular disorders. *Journal of Orofacial Pain, 15*(1), 47-55.

Carlson, C. R., Sherman, Jeffrey J., Studts, Jamie L. &Bertrand, P. L. (1997). The effects of tongue position on mandibular muscle activity. *Journal of Orofacial Pain, 11*, 291-297.

Chaplin, Tara, Cole, Pamela & Zahn-Waxler, Carolyn (2005). Parental socialization of emotion expression. *Emotion, 5* (1), 80-88.

Craske, Michelle G. (2009). *Cognitive-behavioral therapy.* Washington, DC: *American Psychological Association.*

Dittmann, Melissa. (2003). Anger across the gender divide. *Monitor on Psychology, 34* (3), 34, 52.

Dworkin, Sam. (2010). Research diagnostic criteria for temporo-mandibular disorders: Current status and future relevance. *Journal of Oral Rehabilitation, 37*(10), 734–743.

Fillingim, R., Hastie, B., Ness, T., Glover, T., Campbell, C. & Staud, R. (2005). Sex-related psychological predictors of baseline pain perception and analgesic responses to Pentazocine. *Biological Psychology, 69,* 97-112.

Galdas, P., Cheater F., & Marshall P. (2005). Men and health help-seeking behaviour: Literature review. *Journal of Advanced Nursing, 49*(6), 616-23.

Goulet, J., Lavigne, J., & Lund, J. (1995). Jaw pain prevalence among French-speaking Canadians in Quebec and related symptoms of temporomandibular disorders. *Journal of Dental Research, 74*(11),1738-1744.

Jensen, R., Rasmussen, B., Pederson, B., Lous, L. & Olesen, J. (1993). Prevalence of oromandibular dysfunction in a general population. *Journal of Orofacial Pain, 7*(2), 175-82.

Kraus, Hans. (1965). *The Cause, prevention and treatment of backache, stress and tension.* NY: Simon & Schuster.

Laskin, Dan & Greene, Charles. (1972). Influence of the doctor-patient relationship on placebo therapy for patients with myofascial pain dysfunction (MPD) syndrome. *The Journal of the American Dental Association, 85,* 892.

Laskin D. M. (1969). Etiology of the pain-dysfunction syndrome. *The Journal of the American Dental Association, 79*(1),147-153.

Lavigne, Gilles, Sessle, Barry, Choiniere, Manon, & Soja, Peter. (2007). *Sleep and pain.* Seattle, WA: International Association for the Study of Pain.

Legato, Marianne. (2008). *Why men die first: How to lengthen your lifespan.* NY: Palgrave Macmillan.

De Leeuw, Reny. (Ed). (2008). *Orofacial pain: Guidelines for assessment, diagnosis and management,* 4th Edition. IL: Quintessence Publishing.

Lipton, J., Ship, J., & Larach-Robinson, D. (1993). Estimated prevalence and distribution of reported orofacial pain in the U. S. *The Journal of the American Dental Association, 124,* 115-121.

McMillan, A., Wong, M. & Zheng, J. (2006). Prevalence of orofacial pain and treatment seeking in Hong Kong Chinese. *Journal of Orofacial Pain, 20*(3), 218-25.

Mense, S. (2003). The pathogenesis of muscle pain. *Current Pain & Headache Reports, 7*(6), 419-425.

Murphy, Eamonn. (2008). *Managing orofacial pain in practice.* IL: Quintessence Publishing.

Osler Symposia, The. (2011). http://www.oslersymposia.org/about-Sir-William-Osler.html.

Okeson, Jeffrey P. (1995). *Bell's orofacial pains.* IL: Quintessence Publishing.

Pilkey, Ryan. (2011). Why men don't visit the doctor. *Advance for Nurses.* http://nursing.advanceweb.com/Regional-Content/Articles/Why-Men-Dont-Visit-the-Doctor.aspx

Sarno, John. (2006). *The divided mind: The epidemic of mindbody disorders.* NY: HarperCollins.

_____(1991). *Healing back pain: The mind-body connection.* NY: Wellness Central/Hachette Book Group.

_____ (1984) *Mind over back pain.* NY: William Morrow & Co.

Schmidt, John E., Carlson, Charles R., Usery, Andrew R., & Quevedo, Alexandre S. (2009). Effects of tongue position on mandibular muscle activity and heart rate function. *Oral Surgery, Oral Medicine, Oral Pathology, Oral Radiology and Endodontology, 108*(6), 881-888.

Schwartz, Mark S. & Adrasik, Frank. (2003). *Biofeedback: A practitioner's guide,* 3$^{rd}$ edition. New York: Gilford Press.

Seilgman, D. & Pullinger, A. (1991). The Role of intercuspal occlusal relationships in temporomandibular disorders: A review. *Journal of Craniomandibular Disorders, 5,* 96-106.

Simons, David, Simons, Lois & Travell, Janet. 1983). *Myofascial pain and dysfunction: The trigger point manual.* Phila., PA: Lippincott, Williams and Wilkins.

Smith, M. & Haythornthwaite, J. (2004). "How do sleep disturbance and chronic pain inter-relate? Insights from the longitudinal and cognitive-behavioral clinical trials literature. *Sleep Medicine Reviews, 8*(2), 119-32.

Sognnaes, Reidar F. (1977). Why mouthless medical schools? *New England Journal of Medicine, 297,* 837-838.

# DIRECTORY OF HELPING ORGANIZATIONS

If you are seeking more information about facial pain, you can contact any of the following organizations on the Internet for more information, advice, or guidance.

*

American Academy of Orofacial Pain: http://www.aaop.org/

American Headache Society: http://www.americanheadachesociety.org/

International Association for the Study of Pain: http://www.iasp-pain.org/

TNA: Facial Pain Association: http://www.endthepain.org

American Pain Society: http://www.ampainsoc.org/

American Academy of Pain Management: http://www.aapainmanage.org/

European Academy of Craniomandibular Disorders:
http://www.eacmd.org

Ibero Latin American Academy of Orofacial Pain:
(English): http://www.aildc.org/
(Spanish): http://www.aildc.net/

National Institutes of Health: http://www.nih.gov/

# AUTHOR BIOGRAPHIES

## Donald R. Tanenbaum, DDS, MPH

While pursuing a dual degree in Dentistry and Public Health at Columbia University (DDS/MPH) in New York City, Dr. Tanenbaum envisioned a career that would focus on helping patients with facial pain problems. Following a 2-year dental residency at Queens Hospital Center in New York City, where he learned the essentials of the diagnosis and management of chronic benign pain of the head, face and mouth, Dr. Tanenbaum started his professional career. Over the last 26 years he has maintained private practices in New York City and Long Island and devoted countless hours to teaching dental students, dental residents and practicing dentists throughout the United States.

Dr. Tanenbaum holds several prominent positions, including Clinical Assistant Professor at the School of Dental Medicine at the State University of New York at Stony Brook, Clinical Assistant Professor at the North Shore-LIJ School of Medicine at Hofstra University, and Section Head of the Division of Orofacial Pain/Dental Sleep Medicine at the Long Island Jewish Medical Center. Dr. Tanenbaum is a past president of the American Academy of Orofacial Pain, a Fellow of the American Academy of Orofacial Pain, and a Diplomate of the American Board of Orofacial Pain. He has given lectures at medical grand rounds, dental societies and study clubs, and continues to pursue training and education in this specialized area of pain.

## S. L. Roistacher, DDS, FACD, FICD

A pioneer in the field of facial pain, Dr. Seymour Roistacher is a founding member of the International Association for the Study of Pain and the American Pain Society. For over 30 years, he was chair of the Department of Dental Medicine at Queens Hospital Center in New York City and chair of the committee on chronic headache pain. Because of Dr. Roistacher's groundbreaking work and unusual success with chronic pain patients, he became the person to whom the medical staff would turn when their best efforts to deal with major headache and facial pain failed. Dr. Roistacher often conducted grand rounds on the diagnosis and management of chronic benign pain of the head, face and mouth for the departments of internal medicine, otolaryngology, and neurology.

Dr. Roistacher has held numerous faculty appointments, including Clinical Professor of Dentistry, Columbia University School of Dental Medicine; Professor of Dental Medicine, State University of New York at Stony Brook; and Professor of Dentistry, Mt. Sinai School of Medicine. As a member of the American Dental Association's Committee on Graduate Dental Education, he succeeded in having the science, identification, and care of chronic benign headache included in the requirements for approval of dental residency programs. Dr. Roistacher has also written many articles on the diagnosis and treatment of facial pain for numerous medical journals, including the *Journal of Oral Medicine*, the *Journal of Dental Education*, and the *Clinical Journal of Pain*.

# INDEX

head, 6-9, 11, 13, 35-36, 43, 50, 53, 63, 69, 93-96, 110, 114-116
headache, 7, 21, 26, 72, 84, 107, 113, 122
hormones, 21, 59, 62, 95,
hypoxia (oxygen depletion), 60, 69,

immune systems, 17, 58-59
inflammation, 21, 52, 59, 99-102
injury, 1, 3, 12, 16, 25, 34, 53, 64, 71, 75, 87, 100
International Association for the Study of Pain (IASP), 3, 122,
internists, 1, 10

jaw, 1, 4, 6-15, 17-20, 22-23, 33-34, 38-43, 45-52, 55-63, 65-66, 68, 75-76, 78-82, 84, 89-91, 93, 97, 100-101, 103-103, 107, 110-115, 117
    jaw pain, 12, 62, 65, 76, 79-80, 111-112, 115

Kraus, Hans, 13, 120

Legato, Marianne, 21, 120
ligaments, 12, 35-36, 38, 42-43, 48-49, 58-59
lips, 6, 8, 11, 13, 93-96, 108, 111
"long distance runners" (*see "muscles"*)
loss of control, 4, 20, 55, 89

masseter muscle (*see "muscles"*)
medications, 17, 28, 52, 66, 71, 74, 77, 82, 84, 91-92, 99, 114-115
    ADHD, 85
    anti-anxiety, 83, 105
    anti-inflammatory, 99-100
    Botox, 103
    homeopathic remedies, 102
    muscle injections
    muscle relaxants, 5, 100-101
    natural supplements, 102
    nerve sensitization, 101
    pain, 5, 24, 29, 99
    sleep, 102
    topical, 101-102
    transdermal, 101-102
men, 19, 21-23, 26, 33, 54, 112
migraines, 1, 52, 83
*Mind Over Back Pain* (Sarno, 1984), 3, 121

mind-body, 3, 36, 51, 58, 71, 81-82, 88, 92, 96, 105, 118
misdiagnose, 13, 29, 32
misdiagnosis, 18, 29, 32-33
mobility, 9
motor expression, 10-11, 18, 60
mouth, 38-39, 41, 45-46, 48, 53, 64-65, 83, 89, 94-95, 97, 109-114
multiple symptoms, 11, 76
muscles:
    and the "brain under siege," 35-69
    guarding, 63-65, 92
    "long distance runners," 43, 47, 50, 68
    masseter, 15, 114,
    neck (cervical), 36, 44, 50-53, 56, 61-63, 66, 80-81, 93, 98, 103-104, 110
    of mastication, 36-37, 45-46, 49
    "sprinters," 43-47, 50, 68
    sternocleidomastoid, 14, 98
    trapezius, 14, 98
musculoskeletal, xi, 21, 85

nerves, 7, 25, 35-36, 38, 42, 49, 58-60, 62-65, 67, 101, 111
    trigeminal, 60, 63, 111, 115
    vagus, 60
neural expression, 10-11, 18, 60
neuralgia, 1, 28, 110-111, 116
    trigeminal, 28, 108, 111-112
neurologist, 1-2, 10, 20, 28-29, 34, 52, 70, 83, 109
nose, 2, 6, 10, 13, 29, 57, 94-95, 98, 116
numb, 9, 32
numbness, 10-11, 50-51, 60, 63, 110

odd sensations, 9-10, 18, 34
Olsson, Kurt ("Emotional Motor Center"), 54, 57
oral appliances ("nightguards"), 5, 82, 92, 103-104
orofacial pain, xii, 2, 117, 122-123
orofacial pain doctor, 2
Osler, William, 19, 74, 121
otolaryngologists, 1-2, 52, 109, 124
oxygen, 22, 32, 40-41, 45, 51, 59-60, 63-64, 67, 69, 95, 104

pain management, xi-xii, 2, 122
pain patterns, 9-18

126